A Holistic Approach To Arthritis & Management of Chronic Pain

A Holistic Approach To Arthritis
& Management of
Chronic Pain

By

Dr. M.K. Sharma
Pragya Sharma

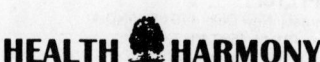

HEALTH HARMONY

An imprint of
B. Jain Publishers (P) Ltd.
USA — EUROPE — INDIA

A HOLISTIC APPROACH TO ARTHRITIS

First Edition: 2000
4th Impression: 2014

NOTE FROM THE PUBLISHERS
Any information given in this book is not intended to be taken as a replacement for medical advice. Any person with a condition requiring medical attention should consult a qualified practitioner or therapist.

All rights reserved. No part of this book may be reproduced, stored in a retrieval system or transmitted, in any form or by any means, mechanical, photocopying, recording or otherwise, without any prior written permission of the publishers.

© with the publishers

Published by Kuldeep Jain for

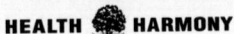

An Imprint of
B. JAIN PUBLISHERS (P) LTD.
1921/10, Chuna Mandi, Paharganj, New Delhi 110 055 (INDIA)
Tel.: +91-11-4567 1000   Fax: +91-11-4567 1010
Email: info@bjain.com   Website: **www.bjain.com**

Printed in India by
JJ Imprints Pvt. Ltd.

ISBN: 978-81-319-0003-1

FOREWORD

*A*rthritis is one of the most common and wide spread diseases of old age known to mankind from time immemorial. Usually the joints of knees, wrists, elbows, fingers, toes, shoulders, hips as well as spine are affected by it. Rain, stiffness, swelling and ultimate disability are the visual symptoms of this disease.

Many forms of arthritis such as gout, ankylosing spondilitis, osteo arthritis and rheumatoid arthritis are genetically transferred in families. Other factors causing arthritis include injury & infection of the joints and auto immune reaction. Hence the factors responsible for the disease may be categorized as heredity and environmental. Further the process of evolution is also responsible for common occurrence of arthritis. Different parts of body especially the skeletons have not yet adjusted to the upright posture and twolegged existence of the species Homo sapiens. This is also one of the reasons that arthritis of neck, back and other weight bearing joints like hips, knees and feet are more common.

In conventional medicine non-steroidal anti-inflammatory drugs and painkillers are most commonly used medicines for arthritis complains. These drugs in a number of cases cause drowsiness, constipation, stomach irritation, ulcers & bleeding. Recently 'designer chaser drugs' have been introduced, which counteract the side effects of other drugs. However, there is no magic cure for this disease as yet.

More and more people are now aware that there are alternative healing methods available. They would like to explore the possibilities but do not know which of these therapies would be suitable for them.

'A HOLISTIC APPROACH TO ARTHRITIS AND MANAGEMENT OF CHRONIC PAIN' is a sincere effort to help people in the field of complementary therapies. The book deals with the functioning of joints and different arthritis disorders in simple terms. It enables the reader to understand the disease and explains the characteristics and limitations of different forms of therapies for persons suffering from arthritis. It also deals in a splendid way the management of the disease and the accompanying pain. The monograph is unique as it deals with synthesis of different systems of medicine e.g. Allopathy, Ayurvedic, Accupressure and Yoga in the management of Rheumatic disorders.

The authors deserve credit for this praiseworthy monograph. This will be a boon to the pharmaceuticals already marketing Ayurvedic and Homeopathic medicines that are widely used in clinical practice.

I strongly recommend the monograph to all health care workers caring for persons afflicted with arthritis and chronic pain of multi-factorial aetiology.

Dr. K. C. Prasad
M.D., FICP, FIAMS
Former Professor & Head of Medicine
Rajendra Medical College, Ranchi
BIHAR

FOREWORD

*R*heumatology refers to the study of medical disorders of joints and connective tissues. These disorders include pain, inflammation and stiffness of joints as well as other supporting elements of muscular skeletal system.

The magnitude of problem is so great that arthritis itself is one of the major causes of disability especially among the elderly. With the enhancement of medical care and awareness, the life expectancy of an average Indian has increased. This has resulted in increased occurrence of joint problems. The various forms of arthritis and its management have been dealt comprehensively in this monograph.

The authors have emphasized the benefits and limitations of different disciplines of medical system e.g. Allopathic, Ayurvedic, Homeopathic, Accupressure and physiotherapy under the heading of Yoga. This difficult subject has been discussed in a common man's language and in a very interesting way.

This monograph *'A HOLISTIC APPROACH TO ARTHRITIS & MANAGEMENT OF CHRONIC PAIN'* will be of immense help to patients having arthritis, their friends and relatives.

Dr. M. K. Govil
M.D., FICA

Former Professor of Medicine,
G. S. V. M. Medical College, Kanpur &
Director, Professor and Head, Deptt. Of Medicine,
Medical College, Allahabad

PREFACE

Arthritis affects approximately 5-10 percent of adult population in India. In elderly people especially in those after fifty years of age, its incidence varies from 15 to 20%. A large number of people need daily medication and many of them consult medical practitioners regularly. However, a large majority suffers in pain silently as they do not have means to get regular medical attention.

In arthritis there is chronic pain, inflammation and stiffness in joints. The intensity and severity of pain varies from time to time but it reminds you its presence all the time. There are large numbers of drugs, which have been invented and marketed by industry in different systems of medicine. As a result there are enormous commercial interests providing services and products to cure the disease and accompanying pain. This raises hopes and as a result you may spend a fortune to find cure, which might not be there.

This book is primarily written for people suffering from arthritis, their relatives and friends. This, however, does not preclude other people to read it as they would find it very interesting and useful in many ways. There is deliberate repetition of facts at a number of places, which has been done to make the reader understand the text without referring to other chapters or even sections of the same chapter.

The treatment of pain is usually based on the assumption that the underlying physical cause must be found out and corrected. This approach is useful when we are treating acute pain but when pain becomes chronic as in case of arthritis, the treatment should not be confined to pain only but to the person as a whole i.e. his suffering, his behaviour and the environment around him. After treating all these factors, you will find that pain is not such an obstacle as you think and can be managed successfully.

The best way to manage arthritis is to educate the patient to handle his own handicap and manage his own pain and to teach him how to use various medicines available to the best of his advantage. The doctors must have a clear understanding of patient's conditions and properties, limitations and side effects of all forms of treatment in use. They must be prepared to part with their knowledge and be willing to educate the patients. The patients on their part should be willing to learn and be prepared to take full responsibility of their health and handle their disease themselves intelligently and correctly. They should understand the enormous value of preventive measures and be willing to use alternative systems of medicine, which have been proved to be very useful in controlling chronic pain without side effects.

The book has been written on the insistence and advice of my wife who was benefited immensely in managing her chronic pain by the holistic approach using medical care based on the synthesis of Allopathy and other systems of medicine.

The book has been organised in three chapters. Chapter one deals with causes of arthritis, different arthritic disorders and misconceptions regarding the disease. In chapter two, different systems of medicine viz. Allopathy, Ayurveda, Homoeopathy, Acupressure and Yoga are discussed. The characteristics of different systems and medicines, their limitations and after effects are also discussed here. The last chapter is the synthesis of different systems of medicine. Here plan for the management of chronic pain is given in eleven steps. The remedies discussed and recommended are simple, practical and with in the reach of common men.

I do not claim to have invented anything new in this book but have made a synthesis of different systems of medicine and have arranged the existing knowledge on the subject in such a way that even a layman can fruitfully use it. The remedies recommended are simple and cost effective and hence even those persons who do not have means to get regular medical care can use them. I am confident that this book will immensely benefit persons suffering from arthritis and chronic pain. The relatives and friends of the patients will also find the book equally useful, as they will be in a position to understand the disease, appreciate the sufferings of the patient and his behaviour. The psychological and moral support from relatives and friends will help the patient in better management of his disorder and accompanying pain and his ultimate rehabilitation.

The one common factor that underlines all the alternative systems of medicines described in this book is the belief in the inherent healing power of the body to cure itself. It also brings out the fact that orthodox medicine and complementary therapies are not mutually exclusive as both have a role to play. A judicious use of different types of remedies will go a long way towards promoting the integrated medicine of new millennium.

(Dr. M.K.SHARMA)

PREFACE

It took me more than twenty long years to recognise the culprit, which was slowly making day-to-day life difficult for me. During my student days, I had to stand two to three hours continuously in chemistry practicals. After the practical, unlike other students, I used to feel exhausted with pain in legs. The complains in this regard to my parents used to be brushed aside as they considered me a delicate girl. Later in life I developed chronic pain in sole of one foot, which continued for few years. I also had pain and stiffness in the lumber region. Initially, I did not bother much. At times I contacted doctors who prescribed vitamin B complex capsules and Calcium tablets. In spite of medication the pain and stiffness continued, how ever, its intensity varied from time to time. Slowly my condition deteriorated further and it became difficult for me to stand for a long time at a stretch. Even during cooking I had to sit or lie down a number of times in one session and used to get tired after walking even for a short distance. Blood tests revealed nothing except that haemoglobin in blood was 10 mg% or less. The doctors prescribed iron capsules in addition to calcium and B complex. However, with all this medication neither did my physical condition improve nor the haemoglobin in blood became normal.

Pain and stiffness in lumbar region, continuous heaviness in legs and chronic pain in the sole of one foot made me feel that something was wrong somewhere. Finally, there was a severe pain in the right pelvic joint which radiated through thigh, knee and leg to the foot. I got my pelvic joint X-rayed and the report revealed sclerosis in pelvic joints, right affected more than left. Very earnestly I consulted a orthopaedist who diagnosed arthritis. The doctor suggested painkillers and calcium tablets saying that there is no medicine for this disease in allopathy.

I was thoroughly disappointed and due to restricted mobility started feeling a bit depressed. However, my husband took it as a challenge. He studied other systems of medicine like Ayurveda, Acupressure, Yoga and of course Homeopathy. The study revealed different types of arthritis and many more ways to combat this nagging ailment. The experiments started and after few sessions of acupressure and yoga, I started getting relief in pain. Ayurvedic medicines were taken to control constipation and indigestion. Besides, specific homeopathic medicines based on symptoms were taken. At times when pain was very severe mild painkiller was also used. After taking the above medicines for more than one and a half-year, my condition improved a lot. Now I can stand for a long time, take long train journeys, and can walk briskly for more than half an hour without feeling much fatigue. I have started leading a normal life again. However, I still take following precautions

- Take regularly Ayurvedic preparations for controlling constipation and indigestion.
- Homoeopathic medicines and Accupressure to control

- pain and stiffness of joints.
- Yogic exercises to increase the mobility of joints.
- Avoid certain foods, which aggravate pain etc.

While scanning the literature I discovered that there were a large number of books on arthritis, but there was no work, which deals with different systems of treatment at one place. I advised my husband to write a small monograph on the subject so that other patients can also benefit from his work on the subject. I helped him in writing and correcting the manuscript and finally in preparation of different diagrams.

PRAGYA SHARMA

ACKNOWLEDGEMENTS

The authors express their gratitude to the following persons for going through the manuscript and contributing towards its refinement. These include Dr. A.K.Sinha MBBS DA, Dr. D.K. Srivastava IFS, Shri B.C.Nigam IFS and Shri N.G. Chaubey BFS. The authors are also grateful to their parents Shri H.P.Sharma, Shri R.K. Sharma, Smt. Kusum Sharma and Smt. V.P. Sharma for their constant encouragement and help. The secretarial help provided by Shri Aftabur Rehman and Md. Tawquir Alam is also thankfully acknowledged.

**DR. M.K.SHARMA &
PRAGYA SHARMA**

ABOUT THE AUTHORS

Dr. M.K.Sharma

*D*r. M.K.Sharma completed his master's degree in physics from Indian Institute of Technology, Delhi and obtained Ph.D. in Quantum optics from the same institute. He joined Indian Forest Service in the year 1975 and is presently working as Chief Conservator of Forests in Forest Department, Bihar.

During the year 1985-86, the author suffered from eczema in the palms which continued for 10-12 years aggravating periodically. The disease could not be cured with the help of conventional medicine even after best medical attention. However, the homeopathic treatment cured the ailment within ten days. After this incidence, he studied and practiced alternative systems of medicine and has cured more than one thousand patients of different disorders. Further, he studied Arthritis in depth and helped a large number of persons having this disorder using holistic approach.

Smt. Pragya Sharma

Smt. Pragya Sharma obtained her master's degree in chemistry in first class from Kanpur University in the year 1977. Being a housewife, did not prevent her from pursuing varied interests and pursuits for knowledge. She completed diploma in fine arts. Her interest in the field of healthcare made her probe into the field of nutrition and she successfully completed a certificate course in Food and Nutrition. All these interests and her own experience with Arthritis were the stepping-stones for the creation of this book, which the author thinks will be of great help to the readers.

Contents

Page No.

Chapter - 1 .... *(1)*

ARTHRITIS & ITS DIFFERENT DISORDERS

1.1 **INTRODUCTION** 3
1.2 **STRUCTURE AND FUNCTION OF JOINTS** 5
    Fig - 1 : FACTORS IN ARTHRITIS 6
    Fig - 2 : DIFFERENT TYPES OF JOINTS 6
    Fig - 3 : STRUCTURE OF A JOINT 7

1.3 **MISCONCEPTIONS REGARDING ARTHRITIS AND OTHER ORTHOPAEDIC PROBLEMS** 9
1.4 **ARTHRITIC DISORDERS** 11
    Fig - 4 : DEFORMITY DUE TO OSTEO-ARTHRITIS 14
    Fig - 5 : DEFORMITY DUE TO RHEUMATOID ARTHRITIS 15
    Fig - 6 : JOINTS IN ANKYLOSING SPONDYLITIS 17
    Fig - 7 : JOINTS IN GOUT 19

Chapter - 2 .... *(23)*

TREATMENT OF ARTHRITIS

2.1 **INTRODUCTION** 25
2.2 **ALLOPATHIC SYSTEM OF MEDICINE** 26
2.3 **AYURVEDIC SYSTEM OF MEDICINE:** 29
2.4 **HOMOEOPATHY AND ARTHIRITIS** 40
2.5 **ACUPRESSURE SYSTEM OF MEDICINE** 55
    Fig - 8 : MAIN BONES OF BODY 58
    Fig - 9 : TRANSVERSE SECTION OF BODY 60
    Fig - 10 : ACUPRESSURE POINTS OF DIFFERENT ORGANS IN FEET 60
    Fig - 11 : ACUPRESSURE POINTS OF DIFFERENT ORGANS IN HANDS 63

	Fig - 12 :	POINTS ON THE BACK SIDE OF HANDS AND FEET	66
	Fig - 13 :	POINTS OF VERTEBRAL COLUMN IN FOOT	68
	Fig - 14 :	POINTS OF VERTEBRAL COLUMN IN HANDS	68
	Fig - 15 :	POINTS OF LIVER AND KIDNEYS	69
	Fig - 16 :	POINTS OF STOMACH	70
	Fig - 17 :	POINTS OF SPLEEN	72
	Fig - 18 :	POINTS OF SMALL INTESTINE AND LARGE INTESTINE	73
	Fig - 19 :	POINTS OF GALL BLADDER	75
	Fig - 20 :	POINTS OF BLADDER, GOVERNING VESSEL AND CONCEPTUAL VESSEL	77
	Fig - 21 :	POINTS OF TRIPPLE HEATER	78
	Fig - 22 :	POINTS OF HEART	78
2.6	**YOGA AND MOBILITY OF JOINTS**		**90**
	Fig - 23 :	YOGIC EXCERCISE TO FACILITATE BOWEL MOVEMENT	94
	Fig - 24 :	YOGIC EXERCISES USEFUL IN GASTRIC TROUBLES	96
	Fig - 25A :	YOGIC EXERCISES FOR JOINTS	97
	Fig - 25B :	YOGIC EXERCISES FOR JOINTS	100
	Fig - 26A :	VAJRASANA AND RELATED ASANA	103
	Fig - 26B :	VAJRASANA AND RELATED ASANA	104
	Fig - 27 :	EXERCISES OF BENDING BACKWARD	108
	Fig - 28A :	EXERCISES OF BENDING FORWARD	110
	Fig - 28B :	EXERCISES OF BENDING FORWARD	111
	Fig - 29A :	SURYA NAMASKAR	116
	Fig - 29B :	SURYA NAMASKAR	117
	Fig - 30 :	EXERCISES FOR PRAYER	120
	Fig - 31A :	MISCELLANEOUS EXERCISES	121
	Fig - 31B :	MISCELLANEOUS EXERCISES	122

Chapter - 3 .... (125)

ARTHRITIS AND PAIN MANAGEMENT

3.1	**INTRODUCTION**	**129**
3.2	**DIFFERENT STEPS FOR PAIN MANAGEMENT**	**130**
	Fig - 32A : POSTURES	139
	Fig - 32B : POSTURES	140
	Fig - 32C : POSTURES	142

Chapter - 4 .... (163)

CONCLUSION

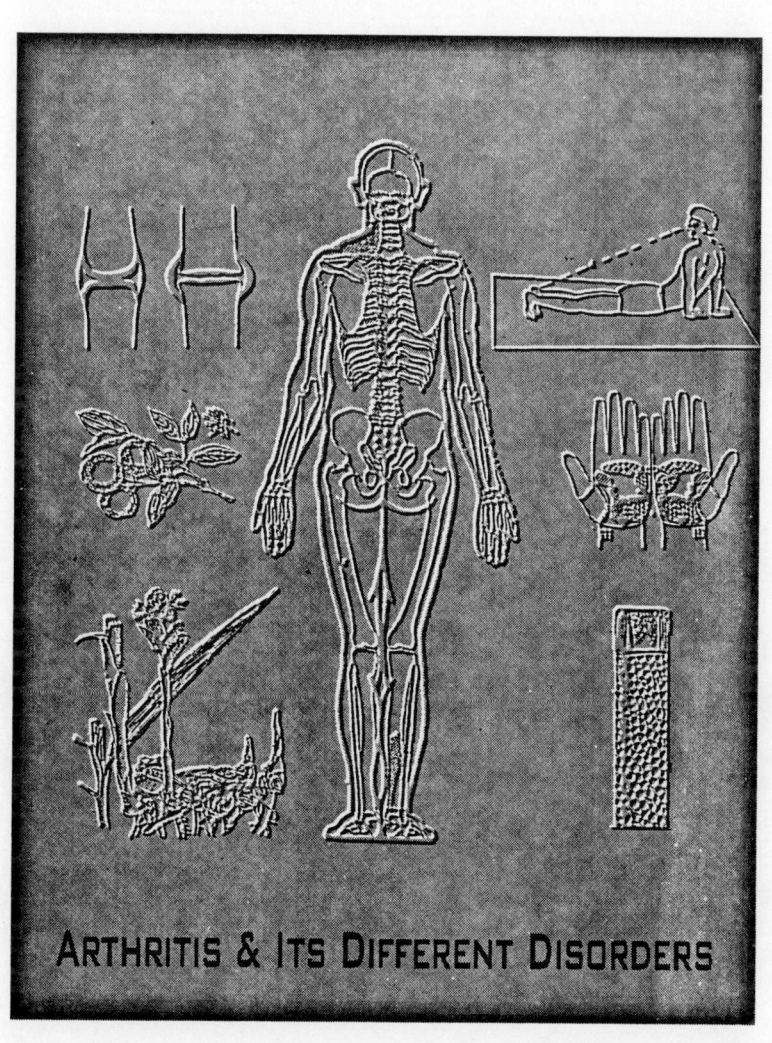

ARTHRITIS & ITS DIFFERENT DISORDERS

Chapter 1

ARTHRITIS & ITS DIFFERENT DISORDERS

1.1 INTRODUCTION

Arthritis is formed from two Greek words i.e. Arthon & itis. Arthon means burning and itis means sensation. Hence there is pain, inflammation and stiffness of joints in arthritis. The joint pain varies enormously in severity from sharp stabbing sensation, burning sensation to grinding pain. In chronic cases there is deformity in one or more joints. Most chronic sufferers find means and ways to cope with pain but pain always exists. Arthritis occurs in knees, wrists, elbows, hips, fingers, toes, shoulders as well as in spine.

The symptoms appear suddenly or gradually; stiffness of joint may be worse in the morning, in the evening or after sitting for a while. In some cases pain is relieved after movement while in other cases movement aggravates. In some cases pain is better by cold applications while in others it is better by warm applications. At times joints get locked momentarily which is caused by weakness of muscles. In some cases movement of joint is badly affected leading to handicap.

As per the allopathic system of medicine, the causes leading to arthritis are not fully understood. Many forms of arthritis are genetically transferred in the family. These include gout, ankylosing spondylitis and to a lesser extent osteo arthritis and rheumatoid arthritis. However, genetics make a person more susceptible to the disease. The arthritis can also be acquired by infection and injury to the joint. (Fig.1)

According to ayurvedic system of medicine different types of diseases in the body are the result of disturbance of equilibrium of vata (air), pitta (bile) and cough. Vata controls respiration, speech, digestion, excretion and nervous system. Pitta controls metabolic process, circulation of blood, digestion and activities of brain. Cough gives nourishment and strength to different parts of the body. It also helps in digestion of food, flexibility of joints and controls secretion of different type of juices from different glands. According to ayurvedic system, the improper functioning of digestive system and disturbed metabolic activity are primarily responsible for arthritis.

Homeopathic system of medicine is based on natural laws of healing. The most important fundamental law of homeopathy is law of similars i.e. like cures the like. This enables the physician to prescribe a remedy based on characteristic symptoms. The homeopaths believe that all parts of body are inter dependent and treat the patient as a whole rather than concentrating on different organs of body separately. The mental and physical illness is treated simultaneously. In the treatment of arthritis, homeopathic system of medicine plays an important part.

In acupressure the disease is treated by applying pressure on specific points with the help of thumb or non pointed object. In arthritis, acupressure has emerged as a consistently better analgesic therapy than any other treatment.

Yoga as a system of medicine also plays an important role in arthritis. Yogic exercises of right kind and proper duration help in reduction of pain and improves mobility of joints. These exercises should be done slowly and increased progressively. These exercises build up muscles and improve mobility of joints. As the muscles are strengthened, the pain is reduced. The mobility of joint is key to the management of pain, resumption of normal activity and finally to rehabilitation. Further exercise stimulates the production of endorphin in the blood stream and increases body's capacity to cope with pain.

In the following paragraphs, we shall discuss structure and function of joints, important types of arthritic disorders and their cure.

1.2 STRUCTURE AND FUNCTION OF JOINTS

The structure of our body makes it possible for many bones to meet with each other and their meeting place is called a joint. The main components of a joint are. (Fig.3)

- Bones
- Cartilages
- Membranes
- Capsules and Ligaments
- Muscles, tendons and bursa
- Fibrous Joints

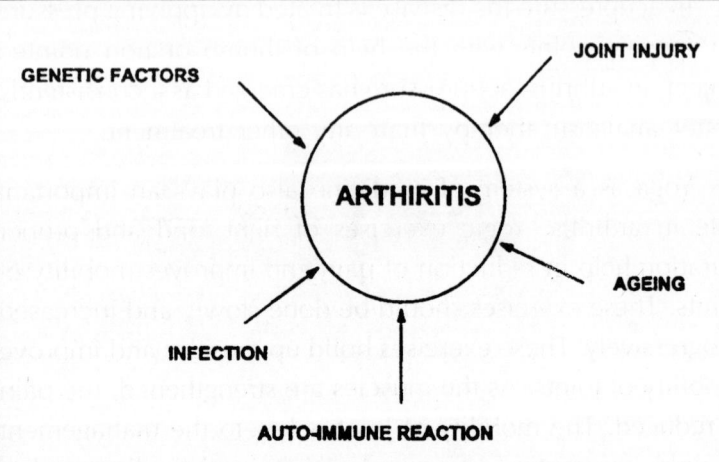

Fig - 1 : FACTORS IN ARTHRITIS

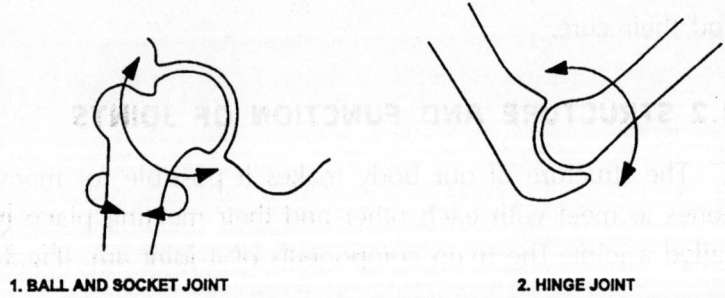

1. BALL AND SOCKET JOINT   2. HINGE JOINT

Fig - 2 : DIFFERENT TYPES OF JOINTS

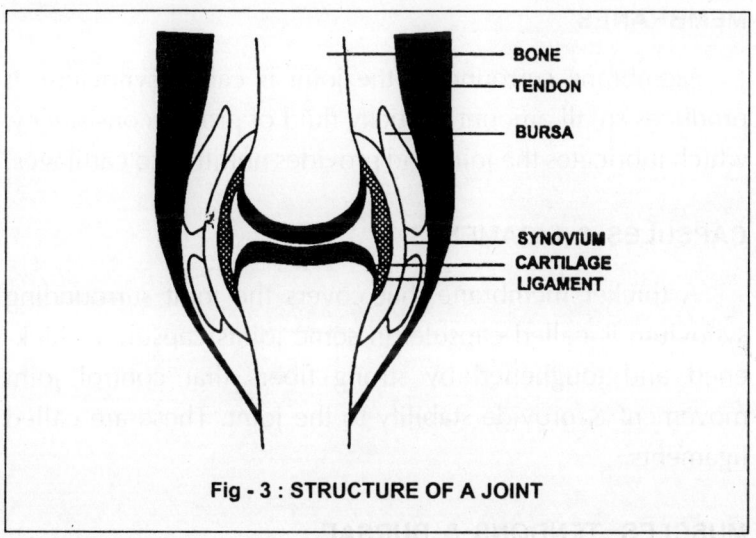

Fig - 3 : STRUCTURE OF A JOINT

BONES

Bones are living tissues. They are made up of calcium phosphate and other minerals. They can change shape or break under abnormal stress. Diseases like arthritis can also damage them. The shape of the bone and type of joint decides the movement. In hinge joints like in elbow, the movement is in one direction only while in case of a ball & socket joint as in hip, the movement is in many directions. (Fig.2)

CARTILAGES

Cartilages are white tissues. They act as shock absorbers and allow smooth movement between two bone ends. Some complex joints like knees have extra pads of cartilage. Cartilages also make up the dishes between the vertebrae. Once damaged, cartilages are usually difficult to be repaired.

MEMBRANES

Membrane surrounding the joint is called synovium. It produces small amount of sticky fluid of proper consistency, which lubricates the joint and provides nutrition to cartilages.

CAPSULES & LIGAMENTS

A thicker membrane that covers the joint surrounding synovium is called capsule. In some joints capsule is thickened and toughened by strong fibers that control joint movement & provide stability to the joint. These are called ligaments.

MUSCLES, TENDONS & BURSAE

Muscles are attached to bones by tendons. There are two types of muscle fibers

- White fibers involved in sudden, jerky & Ill- sustained contractions.
- Red fibers- involved in smooth sustained action. They play an important role in providing better stamina and energy to the muscles. They also provide better flexibility. Yogic exercises strengthen these muscles.

Tendons run over the surface of a joint.

Bursa is a fluid filled sac between tendons and bones. Bursa reduces friction between tendons and bones when they rub against each other. Due to injury tendons and bursa are injured. Like synovium a bursa is prone to inflammation.

FIBROUS JOINTS

Joints in spine, skull and chest consist of a pad of cartilages between bones with no joint cavity. In these joints cartilages act as effective shock absorbers. These joints are called fibrous joints.

1.3 MISCONCEPTIONS REGARDING ARTHRITIS AND OTHER ORTHOPAEDIC PROBLEMS

There are certain misconceptions and preconceived notions about orthopaedic problems. Some of these are

- **Massage Provides Immense Relief In Chronic Pain**

  Massage increases blood circulation in affected part and in turn reduces pain. However, in certain orthopaedic problems massage may aggravate local inflammation and may cause acute muscle spasm.

- **Prolonged Use Of Lumbar Spine Belt And Cervical Collars Are Very Useful**

  Prolonged use of lumbar-spine belt and cervical collar leads to weakening of muscles and stiffness. The collar and belt should be used as per the advice of doctor and not indiscriminately.

- **Persons with Back Pain Should Sleep On A Hard Bed**

  Persons with chronic pain should sleep on a straight rigid bed. Mattresses that are adequately soft and give proper contours are useful. However, very soft mattresses with lumps and irregular patches should be avoided.

- **Persons With Cervical Spondylitis Should Not Use Pillow**

A medium sized pillow, which is comfortable, should be used. A very high pillow should be avoided.

- **Persons with Back Problem Should Never Bend Forward**

Forward bending is restricted in acute phase of prolapsed disc. However, the forward bending muscles are biggest shock absorbers. As the problem gets under control, forward bending is recommended. If these muscles become stiff due to non-use, they will increase load on spine resulting in pain with slightest injury.

- **Persons With Orthopaedic Problem Should Be Given Complete Rest**

Initially for few days the rest is unavoidable. However, care should be taken that rest does not rust the body. Prolonged continuous rest makes the muscles weak and in turn aggravates the problem.

- **Obesity Causes Arthritis**

Obesity does not cause arthritis. However, in people with arthritis, being obese puts more burden on the joints and aggravates the pain.

- **Arthritis Is Caused By Vigorous Exercise**

Vigorous exercise does not cause arthritis. However joint injury or infection may cause arthritis. In case of persons with arthritis, vigorous exercise will aggravate pain.

- **Certain Foods May Cause Arthritis**

Any type of food does not cause arthritis but pain in arthritis is aggravated by certain foods.

- **Too Much Exposure To Cold & Moist Weather Causes Arthritis**

    Arthritis is not caused but pain is aggravated by cold and /or moist conditions.

- **Pain In The Back Or Any Part Of Body Is Due To Arthritis**

    Pain may be due to injury or muscle sprain. Hence, pain in any part of body is not always due to arthritis.

1.4 ARTHRITIC DISORDERS

Though there are more than 200 different types of arthritis, we shall discuss mainly those types of arthritis that are most common & affect more than 90% of people having arthritis. These include osteo-arthritis, rheumatoid arthritis, ankylosing spondylitis, gout, juvenile chronic arthritis and arthritis in elderly people.

OSTEO-ARTHRITIS

It is the most important and most common form of joint disease. It commonly appears in old age after 50. Women are more prone to its attack than men. Aging of joints and genetic configuration make people more prone to this disease. Any severe damage to the joints increases the chances of developing osteo arthritis at that site. Though osteo arthritis is mild but some sufferers have severe joint damage, pain and disability. The joints most often damaged are of knees, hips, and those of hands and feet i.e. base of big toe and thumb and joints at the end of fingers. Some joints in the back are also affected.

SYMPTOMS

Osteo-arthritis starts slowly. Sometimes affected joint gets worse suddenly after minor injury. Pain is the main symptom and is usually worse when joints are being used. There is mild joint stiffness in the morning and sticking of joints after rest and inactivity. Some people have cracking sensation and locking of joints.

At times there is a mild firm swelling at the edges of the damaged joints. There is pain when the joint is moved to the extreme of its range. A special form of arthritis occurs in women around the time of manopause. It starts abruptly with inflammation, heat and redness of joints of fingers. It continues for few years leaving stiff finger joints.

In older people sometimes there is sudden worsening of joints. In such cases there are two possible reasons. The surface of damaged joint suddenly collapses causing severe pain and stiffness. At times calcium crystals formed in the joint gets dislodged causing inflammation with accompanying pain.

OSTEO ARTHRITIS AND REPAIR PROCESS

Normal joints, used normally will never get osteo arthritis however long we live. However if the cartilages and other tissues in the joints are a little weaker than normal and the structure of the joint is such that it puts more stress on the joint or if repair process of the joint is not good, the joint will develop this disorder. (Fig.4) The osteo-arthritis is also developed after fracture of bones, gout or rheumatoid arthritis. This is called secondary osteo-arthritis.

In osteo-arthritis, a battle continues between mechanical factors that cause damage to the joint and the ability of the body to repair it. The thickening of bones and capsules is body's attempt to repair the damage. The repairing process continues in cartilages also. Some times joints may heal but in most of the cases they stabilize after a certain degree of damage.

RHEUMATOID ARTHRITIS

Rheumatoid arthritis causes severe crippling joint damage and a number of other complications. Women are affected more often than men are. It usually begins in early adulthood but in the case of women there is more susceptibility at the time of manopause. If a number of persons in your family have it, you have more chances to get this disease.

What causes rheumatoid arthritis is not properly understood. Rheumatoid arthritis is an auto-immune phenomenon. It means that the immune system, which normally defends us against infections, attacks the joints. It is the abnormal immune reaction that keeps this disease going.

SYMPTOMS

The synovium gets inflamed, swollen, red and hot. Excess fluid and cells leak out of synovium and the whole joint becomes swollen and painful. The inflammation can occur in tendons as well as bursae which causes pain during movement. Some people develop nodules, which are patches of inflammation. Sometimes lining of the heart, eyes, nerves, blood vessels in skin and even kidneys are affected. In rheumatoid arthritis, inflammation in the joint continues for

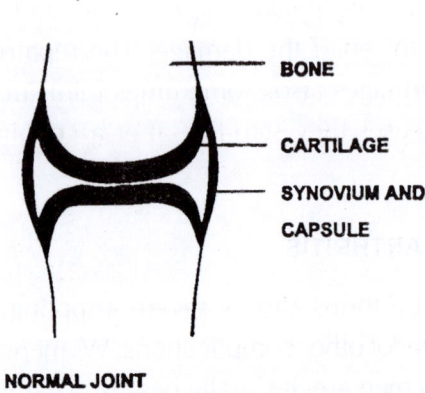

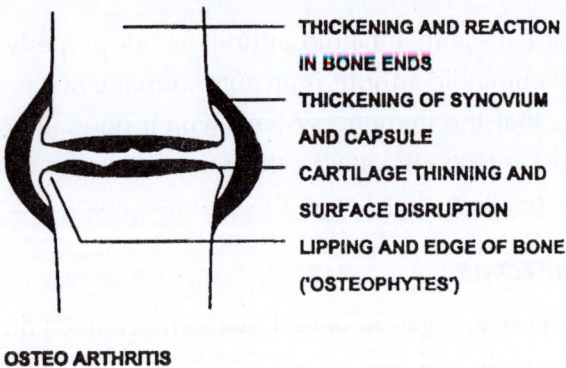

Fig -4 : DEFORMITY DUE TO OSTEO-ARTHRITIS

Arthritis & Its Different Disorders

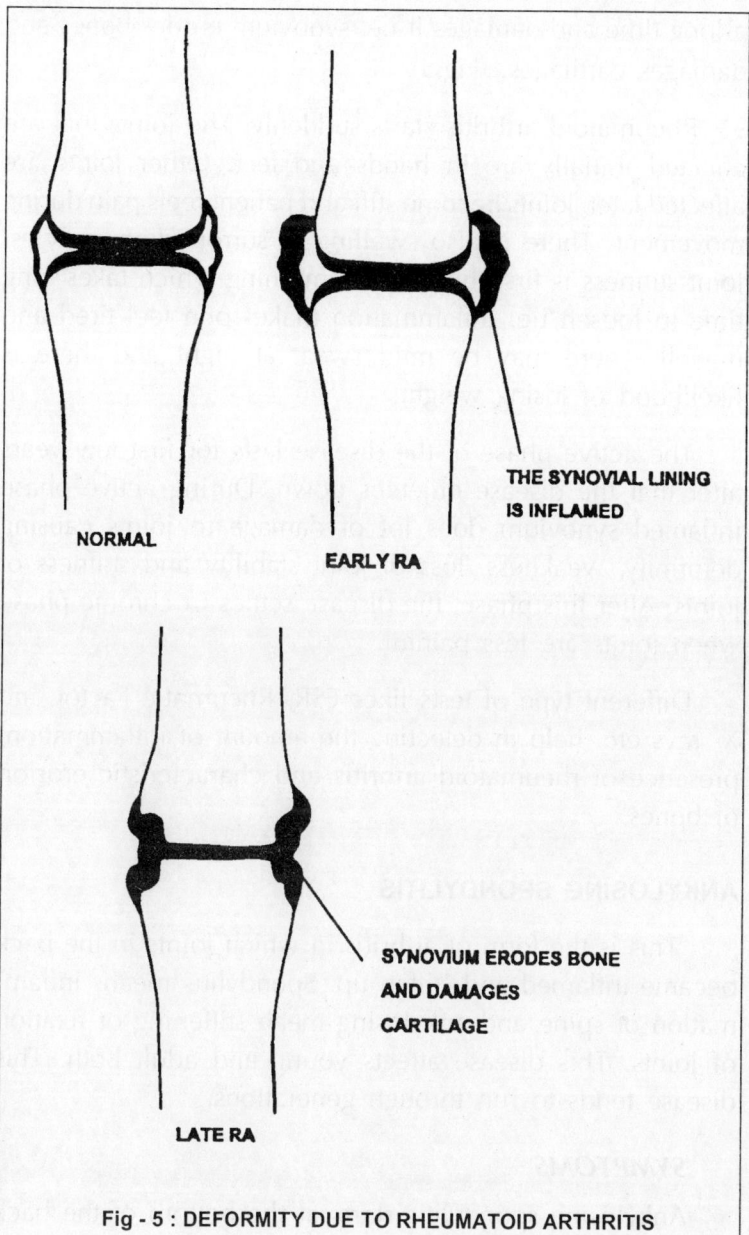

NORMAL

EARLY RA

THE SYNOVIAL LINING IS INFLAMED

LATE RA

SYNOVIUM ERODES BONE AND DAMAGES CARTILAGE

Fig - 5 : DEFORMITY DUE TO RHEUMATOID ARTHRITIS

a long time and damages it i.e. synovium erodes bones and damages cartilages. (Fig.5)

Rheumatoid arthritis starts suddenly. The joints that are affected initially are in hands and feet. Other joints are affected later. Joints become stiff and patient feels pain during movement. There is also swelling in surrounding muscles. Joint stiffness is first thing in the morning which takes long time to loosen up. Inflammation makes one feel tired and unwell. There may be mild sweat at night and there is likelihood of losing weight.

The active phase of the disease lasts for first few years after that the disease quietens down. During active phase inflamed synovium does lot of damage to joints causing deformity, weakness, loss of joint stability and stiffness of joints. After this phase, the disease settles in chronic phase when joints are less painful.

Different type of tests likes ESR, Rheumatic Factor and X- rays etc. help in detecting the amount of inflammation, presence of rheumatoid arthritis and characteristic erosion of bones.

ANKYLOSING SPONDYLITIS

This is the form of arthritis in which joints in the back became inflamed and stiffen up. Spondylitis means inflammation of spine and ankylosing mean stiffening or fixation of joints. This disease affects young and adult both. This disease tends to run through generations.

SYMPTOMS

Ankylosing spondylitis starts at the bottom of the back and travels up the spine within few years. In few patients,

Arthritis & Its Different Disorders

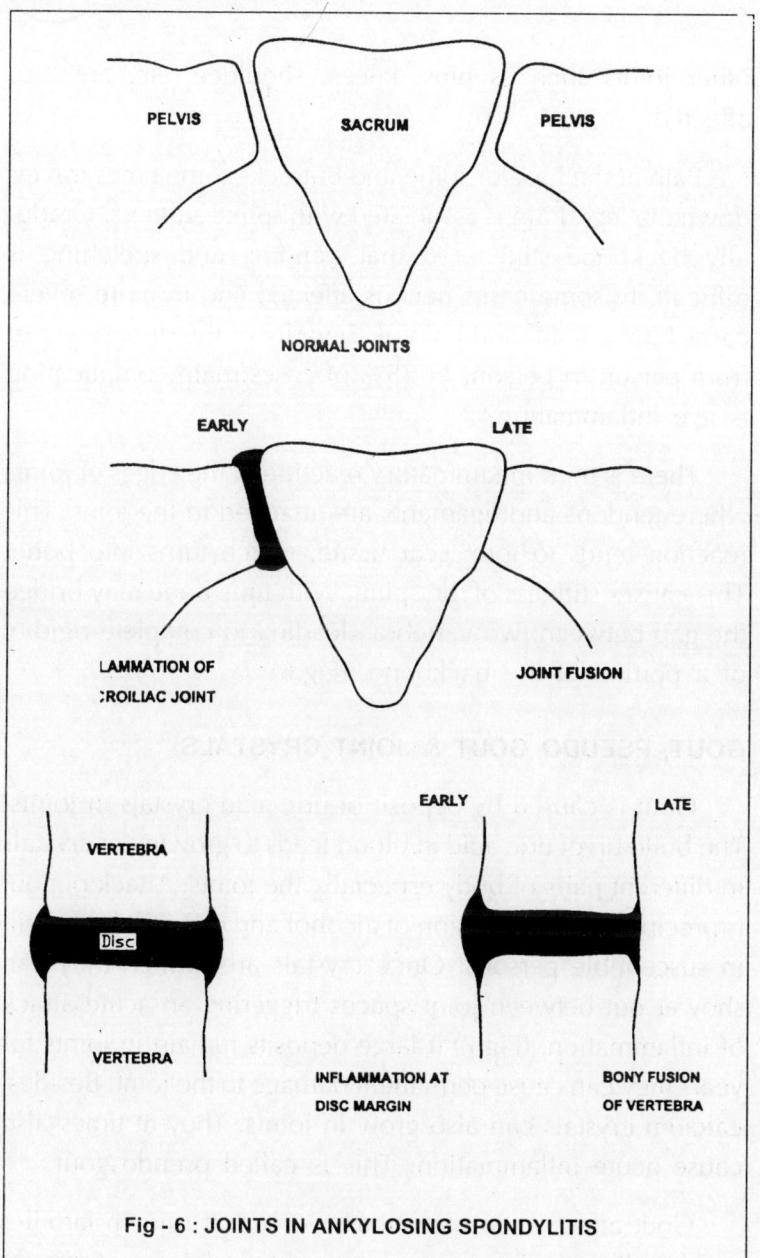

Fig - 6 : JOINTS IN ANKYLOSING SPONDYLITIS

other joints such as hips, knees, shoulders etc. are also affected.

Pain at the base of spine and buttocks some times travels down the legs. Pain is associated with spinal stiffness. Gradually backbone stiffens so that bending and stretching is difficult. In some cases neck is affected and in more severe cases hips get stiff and painful. Severity of the disease varies from person to person. In 25% of cases main complication is eye inflammation.

There is mild inflammatory reaction at the edges of joints where tendons and ligaments are attached to the joint. This reaction tends to form scar tissue, which turns into bone. This causes stiffness of the spine. With time bone may bridge the gap between two vertebrae leading to complete rigidity of a portion of the backbone. (Fig.6)

GOUT, PSEUDO GOUT & JOINT CRYSTALS

Gout is caused by deposit of uric acid crystals in joints. The build up of uric acid in blood leads to growing of crystals in different parts of body especially the joints. Attack of gout is precipitated by ingestion of alcohol and diet rich in protein in susceptible persons. Once crystals are formed they can shower out between joint spaces triggering an acute attack of inflammation. (Fig.7) If large deposits remain in joints for years they can cause permanent damage to the joint. Besides, calcium crystals can also grow in joints. They at times also cause acute inflammation. This is called pseudo gout.

Gout affects men more than women. It runs in families and usually starts in young adulthood & middle age. Sufferers are often overweight.

SYMPTOMS

Gout usually starts with an acute attack mostly at the base of the big toe. Usually it starts with no apparent reason. Toe becomes red, swollen and extremely painful. Other parts such as foot, ankle, hand, wrist, knee, or elbow are also affected. The duration of attack varies. Long lasting gout may lead to kidney stones and kidney damage.

Blood test as well as test of fluid from the joint can detect gout.

Gout sufferers should keep fit, avoid cigarettes, alcohol and diet rich in protein. For obese people, simply losing little weight will help reduce the amount of uric acid in blood sufficiently. In some elderly people, growth of crystals in joint cartilages contributes to the development of osteo arthritis.

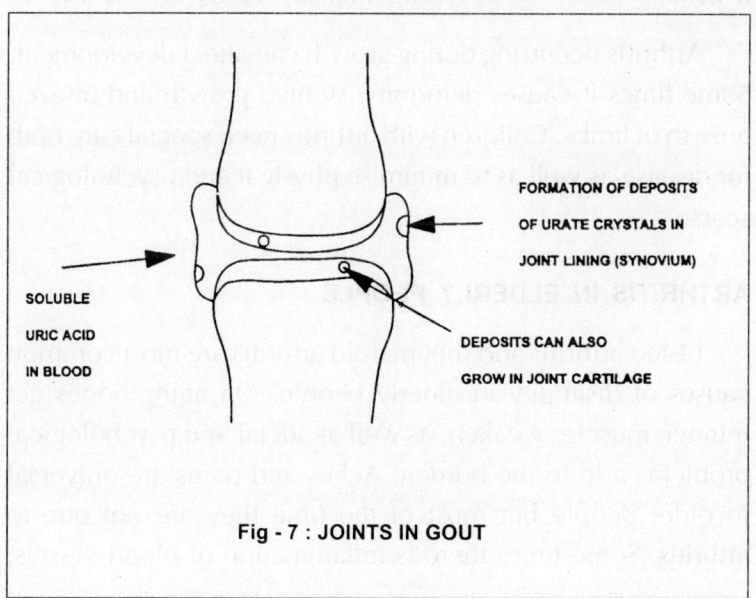

Fig - 7 : JOINTS IN GOUT

ARTHRITIS IN CHILDHOOD

Joint pains are common in children. Viral infection is a common cause of short lasting muscle and joint pains. Besides, injury and eccessive exercise are other causes of joint pain.

There are small numbers of arthritic diseases in children. Most childhood arthritis seen today is known as juvenile chronic arthritis. This is the condition of pain and swelling of one and more joints that persists for more than three months in children under 16 years of age. The commonest type affects a number of joints. Another type is like rheumatoid arthritis which causes wide spread joint damage. Yet another type causes fever & rashes. It is a manifestation of rheumatic heart disease that affects mainly bigger joints of the body e.g. knee joint, ankle joint and elbow joint. It usually follows 4-6 weeks after an attack of sore throat.

Arthritis occurring during growth can affect development. Some times it causes deformity, stunted growth and uneven growth of limbs. Children with arthritis need special care both for disease as well as to minimise physical and psychological scars.

ARTHRITIS IN ELDERLY PEOPLE

Osteo arthritis and rheumatoid arthritis are most common causes of disability in elderly people. On aging bones get thinner, muscles weaken, as well as social and psychological problems add to the burden. Aches and pains are universal in older people but most of the time they are not due to arthritis. Some times there is inflammation of blood vessels, which occasionally causes strokes and blindness. It is called **polymyalgia rheumatica**. However, this disease responds quickly to small doses of steroid tablets.

■ ■

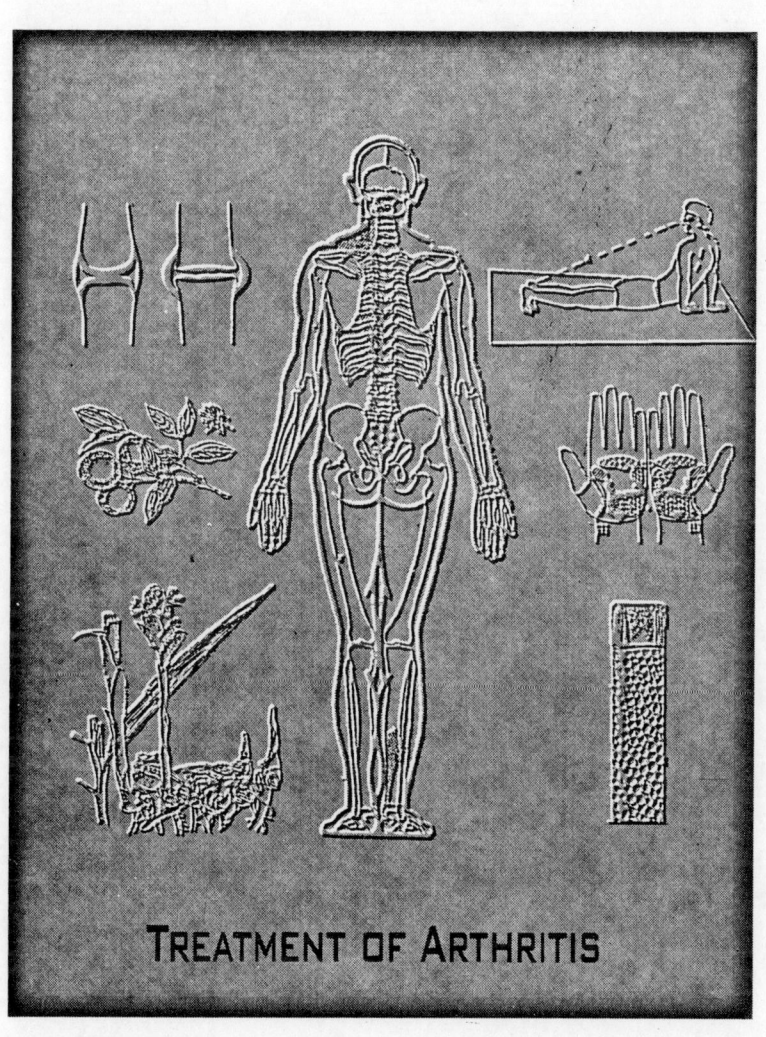

TREATMENT OF ARTHRITIS

Chapter

2

TREATMENT OF ARTHRITIS

2.1 INTRODUCTION

In the treatment of chronic pain the focus is on pain management. It is based on the understanding that pain is not merely a physical problem. It enables the patient to receive a variety of treatment i.e. medical, psychological as well as complementary medicine. Over and above this, it teaches the patients the skills to help themselves and to accept the fact that managing pain is a full time occupation and is a pre-requisite to enjoyment of better quality of life. It encourages the patient to change his attitude and become an active participant in his own rehabilitation rather than a passive recipient of medical care. The treatment should not be confined to pain but given to the person so that he is restored physically, mentally and spiritually to cope with every aspect of life while suffering with chronic pain.

Most of the people with chronic pain are written off as hopeless cases. They have physical problems, emotional problems and inter-personal problems. However, it is possible for most of the people to acquire high degree of skill in managing their pain without being dependent on drugs. They can regain mobility, confidence and self- esteem and can contribute positively to the society.

We shall now discuss Allopathic, Ayurvedic, Homeopathic, and Acupressure and Yogic systems of medicine for treatment of arthritis and management of pain.

2.2 ALLOPATHIC SYSTEM OF MEDICINE

INTRODUCTION

In this system of medicine the pain and inflammation in the joint is relieved with the help of painkillers, anti-inflammatory drugs, steroids and injections. The drugs, their uses and side effects are discussed in the following sections.

PAIN KILLERS AND ANTI-INFLAMMATORY DRUGS

Painkillers reduce pain but do not treat the cause of pain. They work by blocking the transmission of pain signals to the brain. On the other hand the anti-inflammatory agents reduce inflammation and by reducing inflammation, they reduce pain. In practice painkillers and anti-inflammatory drugs are used in combination.

Painkillers can cause drowsiness & constipation. Painkillers like morphine are addictive. The anti-inflammatory drugs may cause indigestion and occasionally ulcers, rashes, drowsiness and fluid retention.

Most of the painkillers and anti-inflammatory drugs work only for few hours. It is advisable to limit their use at times when pain is particularly bad and unbearable.

STEROIDS

Steroids including cortisone are a group of body hormones, which affect body's metabolism. In arthritis they are used to reduce inflammation.

Small doses of steroids for a short time can provide relief without side effects. However, extra doses given for a long period can have a number of serious side effects. These include thinning of bones and skin, excess body fat, high blood pressure, cataract and other complications.

INJECTIONS

Special forms of medicines are used for this purpose which when injected into the affected joint stays there and very small quantity gets absorbed into circulation.

The main drugs used are steroids, which reduce inflammation. Acids are used to burn out inflamed tissues. Irradiation is used to reduce arthritic inflammation. Besides, local anaesthetic drugs are also used in combination with above drugs for relief of pain.

DISEASE CONTROLLING AND MODIFYING DRUGS

These drugs slowdown or control the damage. They take a long time to work before the results are visible. When they are effective, there is dramatic improvement in all aspects of disease.

In case of drugs for gout, they reduce uric acid formation in the body. Other group of drugs helps kidneys to increase the amount of uric acid excreted in urine. Similarly drugs for other forms of arthritis also fall in two categories. The first category consist of immune-suppressive agents which include azathioprine and cyclophosphamide etc. The other group cures rheumatoid and other form of arthritis and includes gold, hydroxychloroquine and sulphasalazine etc. These drugs should however be used carefully and their side effects monitored regularly by the doctor.

SURGERY

Decision of opting for surgery is a part of total patient management. It is not a last resort but an important means of treating the disease. If right operation is done at a right time, it will help the patient tremendously.

All types of arthritis do not require surgery. Osteo-arthritis and rheumatoid arthritis when very severe may require surgery. People with ankylosing arthritis may require surgery of spine and hips in rare cases. The percentage of arthritic patients requiring surgery is very small. Surgery can be divided into two types

(a) Peri- articular - Outside joint
(b) Articular - On joint

[a] PERI- ARTICULAR SURGERY

It is relatively minor and includes repair of damaged tendons and ligaments and removal of cysts and nodules.

[b] ARTICULAR SURGERY

- It consists of surgery in which if the synovium is bulky and inflamed and causing mechanical problems, it can be removed. It is called **synovectomy**.

- Bone next to a painful joint is cut and fixed in a different position. It is done to correct deformity and relieve pain in Osteo-arthritis and is called **osteotomy**.
- In a joint, which is restricted in movement and is very painful, is permanently fixed either by nailing or wiring two halves or by bone grafting. It is called **athrodesis**.
- In case of severely damaged joints, **joint replacement surgery** is performed. It can be done on knees, hips, hands, spine, foot, shoulders and elbows etc.

Artificial joints are not perfect and are not as efficient as natural joints. At times lots of complications spoil the success. A good joint replacement provides adequate range of movement for 10-15 years without pain.

2.3 AYURVEDIC SYSTEM OF MEDICINE:

INTRODUCTION

According to ayurvedic system, arthritis is caused by disturbance in digestive system and metabolic activities of the body.

According to ayurvedic science, if a person has constipation, the waste products produced during digestion and the metabolic process of the body, keep accumulating in colon and rectum and water present in the feces gets absorbed in tissues. If the feces do not come out in time, it makes the digestive system weak and the waste products get absorbed in blood. 35% of stool is made up of solid products and about 20 % of it comprise of bacteria. Some bacteria present in colon produce necessary elements for the body. In case of constipation, the harmful bacteria can't come out of body and multiply. They do not allow proper functioning of useful bacteria. The poisonous elements of these harmful bacteria get mixed in blood and affect the metabolic process adversely.

During the process of digestion, in the presence of different enzymes, various reactions take place. As a result of these reactions, gas is formed. The gas generally passes out along with feces. When gas does not come out along with stool due to constipation, the pressure of gas creates lot of trouble in joints.

With chronic constipation all our efforts to relieve pain or cure the disease will not be very successful. The same is true if digestion of food takes unusually long time as in dysentery. One of the most important steps in pain relief is to control constipation as well as improve digestion of food.

METHODS TO CONTROL CONSTIPATION AND INDIGESTION

[a] SET SOLAR PLEXUS IN ORDER

Solar plexus controls functioning of all organs and is situated below diaphragm. Solar plexus shifts upwards or downwards by lifting heavy weight as well as by severe gas trouble. Upward shifting of solar plexus leads to constipation while downward shifting brings indigestion and more motion. Solar plexus can not be set by medicines. Hence before starting any treatment of digestive systems, it is necessary to check the position of solar plexus and set it in order.

METHOD TO KNOW WHETHER SOLAR PLEXUS IS IN ORDER

i. Lie on hard surface and press your finger or thumb in the navel, if you feel throbbing sensation like that of heart, the solar plexus is in order.

ii. If solar plexus is in order, distance between right nipple and navel should be equal to that between left nipple and navel.

iii. Lie down on your back. Keep arms straight on your side. Keep legs straight and toes upright. If two big toes are in level the solar plexus is in order.

BRINGING SOLAR PLEXUS IN ORDER

i. By putting weight on the navel and trying to push it towards the center. Do it a number of times till by pressing your thumb in the navel throbbing sensation is felt.

ii. Lie down on your back. Exhale the breath fully. Now inhale and inflate the stomach as much as possible and keep it as long as you cán. Repeat it till solar plexus is in order.

iii. Put a small oil lamp on navel, cover it with metal glass, hold it for some time till oxygen is burnt out and there is vacuum. Vacuum will bring solar plexus in order. Now lift the glass after one minute. Repeat it till solar plexus is in order.

iv. Lie down on your back with legs straight. Ask some one to put pressure on the knee of the leg (of which big toe is at lower level) and simultaneously pull up the big toe which is lower.

[b] DIET

INTRODUCTION

There is a strong relationship between intake of food and development and cure of diseases. The diet also has an impact on immune system and diseases such as arthritis, osteoporosis etc. Improving the quality of diet and supplementing it with immune boosting substances can help reduce pain and inflammation.

We need nutrients in correct amount for good health. Nature has packed unprocessed food with nutrients, minerals and vitamins. The vitamins are delicate and unstable entities that can easily be destroyed during processing of food. The food is depleted of vitamins and minerals in the process of its progress from farm to factory, factory to market, market to freezer/oven and then on to the plate. One should therefore avoid tinned, processed and preserved food.

For healthy bones and joints the diet should consist of foods that are low in fats, high in fiber content and have adequate level of vitamins and minerals. In case of deficiency of vitamins and minerals, supplements may be taken in consultation with nutritionalist. Large doses of supplements are inefficient and may cause deficiency of other nutrients. The vitamins and mineral intake supplement each other. Vitamin C is necessary for the absorption of iron, vitamin D and magnesium are necessary for the utilization of calcium and vitamin E protects vitamin A and D from oxidation. Sometimes large quantities of some nutrients deplete others e.g. large quantities of zinc can deplete copper, creating an imbalance of system.

- *Acid/Alkali Balance in Diet*

Acid /alkali balance is very important in controlling inflammatory condition. The diet that is predominantly alkaline would help in reducing inflammation. However, the dietary need is different for each individual. In general a diet consisting of 75% alkali forming foods and 25% acid forming foods is an ideal balance. Most foods and vegetables except citrus fruits and tomatoes are alkali forming. Other acid forming foods are dairy foods, meat, fish and most cereals.

In order to control inflammation and keep digestive system in order, the following diet and everyday routine should be followed.

- **FIX A MEAL SCHEDULE AND STICK TO IT:**

In order to ensure regular bowel movement, fix a time schedule for food and stick to it. Do not take food at odd hours or in hurry. Do not take food when you are not feeling hungry.

- **CHEW FOOD WELL:**

By chewing food well, adequate quantity of salivary juices are mixed with food, which help in its digestion. Avoid taking food while watching TV, listening to radio, reading newspaper or during movement.

- **GRAINS:**

Whole grain wheat flour and unpolished rice should be used. Barley, maize, jowar and millets are helpful in controlling constipation.

- **MILK AND MILK PRODUCTS:**

One glass of hot milk taken two hours after night meals

is good for controlling constipation. After the age of 40 years, fat free milk is more useful. Vegetarians should take milk and milk products regularly.

Persons with arthritis should avoid sour curd completely. They can, however, take buttermilk made out of curd, which is not sour. Salt and cumin seeds powder should be mixed with it.

- *VEGETABLES AND FRUITS:*

In case of constipation vegetables are very useful. Patients should take vegetables in greater quantity particularly those with green leaves. The vegetables such as spinach, turnip, gourd, cabbage, brinjal, green papaya, carrot, capsicum, drumsticks etc. are useful. However, one should avoid vegetables, which cause constipation and produce more gas such as lady's fingers, pumpkin, jackfruit, cauliflower & yam etc. Tomato is harmful in arthritis.

Fruit and fruit juice is very effective to prevent constipation. Fresh juice is better than canned juice. Among the fruits ripe papaya, apple, guava etc. are very useful.

Among dry fruits dried grapes berries and figs are useful. Keep them soaked overnight before eating.

- *PULSES:*

Pulses are main source of protein in case of vegetarian people. Besides moong, all other pulses produce gas and cause constipation. They should be taken in less quantity and ghee, garlic, ginger and cumin seeds etc. should be mixed when preparing them.

- **MEAT AND FISH:**

  This food can be taken in very restricted quantity.

- **OILY AND SOUR FOOD:**

  In arthritis one should avoid oily foods. Sour foods should also be avoided. Amla and pomegranate can however be taken, as they are beneficial.

- **STIMULATING DRINKS:**

  Large quantities of tea and coffee cause disorders of digestion and ultimately constipation. Taking tea on empty stomach is very harmful. Liquor taken in large quantity causes cirrhosis of liver. It also affects digestive system adversely. Similarly chewing or smoking tobacco is harmful.

- **SPICES:**

  Green and red chilly are harmful for stomach. But there are some spices, which are very useful for stomach and bowels and give relief in constipation. Black pepper, ginger, cardamom, cinnamon, cloves, cumin seeds and long pepper are very useful. Besides, turmeric is also a good remedy to control constipation.

- **ESSENTIAL VITAMINS AND MINERALS**

  All living beings that use oxygen also produce free radicals i.e. unstable molecules, which lack an electron. These free radicals are kept in check by body's anti-oxidants. However if the body starts making more free radicals than it requires, there is a risk of damage to immune system and of developing chronic diseases.

  As the free radicals are hazardous to health, it is important to neutralize them. Commonly recognized anti-oxidants are vitamin A, vitamin C and vitamin E and minerals zinc and selenium. An imbalance of calcium may cause bones to be porous and more prone to wear and tear.

Different vitamins and minerals useful in arthritis are discussed below.

- *Vitamin A*

Vitamin A is found in eggs, meat, milk, liver oil and dairy products.

- *Vitamin C*

Vitamin C is very important for the formation of both bones and cartilages. It is abundantly found in amla. It is also found in citrus fruits and green vegetables.

- *Vitamin E*

Vitamin E increases oxygen supply to muscles. As an anti-oxidant vitamin E stabilizes membranes and protects them. It protects eyes, skin, liver and calf muscle tissues etc. It increases body's store of vitamin A. It is enhanced by vitamin C and mineral selenium.

Foods rich in vitamin E are nuts, seeds, wheat germ, spinach, broccoli, butter, bananas and strawberries etc.

- *Calcium and Magnesium*

Calcium is most abundant in body, 99% of calcium is present in bones while remaining 1% is found in the muscles, nerves and blood stream. For absorption and proper use of calcium, magnesium and vitamin D are required.

- *Iron*

  In addition to its role in carrying oxygen to cells, iron also performs the function of an anti-oxidant. In inflammatory condition iron level in synovial fluid increases, which indicates that it helps in controlling joint damage.

- *Selenium*

  Inaddition to its role as an anti-oxidant, selenium helps in reducing inflammation.

- *Zinc*

  Zinc is an anti-oxidant. It helps to clear certain toxic materials like cadmium and lead from the body. Zinc is essential for normal cell division. Zinc helps in reducing inflammation and is active in synovial fluid along with iron.

[C] OTHER METHODS TO CONTROL CONSTIPATION:

ENEMA

Enema should only be used in a state of acute constipation. If it is taken regularly, the colon will be inactivated and will not perform its natural function.

PURGATIVES

Persons with chronic constipation generally become dependent on purgatives. Purgatives give quick relief but they also cause several problems and colon becomes fully dependent on it & stops its natural function. Moreover, purgatives produce lesions in inner walls of colon.

TREPHALA

Take one spoon powder of three fruits (powder made from mixing Amla, Bahera and Harra in equal proportion) in one glass of water. Keep it overnight. Next morning filter it with a thin clean piece of cloth and drink it. This helps in controlling constipation, hyper acidity and high blood pressure.

ISAPGOL

Isapgol has been used for centuries in ancient Indian medicine. It has high soluble fiber content and is used to prevent constipation. Regular use of isapgol has also been reported to reduce cholesterol levels.

AYURVEDIC MEDICINE

Ayurvedic medicine is extracted from roots, bark, fruits & seeds of different trees, shrubs & herbs. In arthritis these medicines are very useful in reducing pain and inflammation of joints. These roots and herbs are either used independently or in combination with other medicines. We shall discuss some important herbs, which are used in the treatment of arthritis.

[a] GINGER (GINGER OFFICINALE)

Ginger root is used as a medicine. It is useful in rheumatoid arthritis, sciatica, cervical spondylitis etc. Ginger can be taken in the form of juice, powder, concentrate or paste.

[b] CASTOR OIL PLANTS (RICINUS COMMUNIS)

Leaves, roots, seeds and their oil are used as medicine. The leaves are boiled in water and application of that water on joint relieves the pain. Castor oil is useful for osteo-arthritis, rheumatoid arthritis, and sciatic and cervical spondylitis. Castor oil is a purgative and is used to clean the stomach. The hot castor oil on application to joint relieves pain.

[c] NUX VOMICA

The bark of this plant along with ripe dried seeds is used as medicine. The seeds of nux vomica are refined and powder is made out of it. This powder is very useful as medicine for osteo-arthritis and rheumatoid arthritis. 100 mg of this powder should be taken twice a day with milk.

[d] GUM GUGGUL (COMMIPORA MUKUL)

It is used as a medicine for osteo-arthritis & rheumatoid arthritis. Two to three year old gum guggul is very useful for reducing cholesterol in blood and controlling obesity. After cleaning guggul, it is mixed with trephala and other medicines and different types of medicines are made out of it e.g. Yograj Guggul, Mahayograj Guggul, Chandra Prabhavati etc. which are very useful in treatment of arthritis.

[e] GARLIC (ALLIUM SATIVUM)

Garlic root is used as a medicine. It is very useful in curing rheumatoid arthritis, sciatica, cervical spondylitis and lumbago etc.

In addition to above roots and herbs, the root & herbs of following plants are also very useful. They include Vitex nigundo, Pluch lanceolata, Poederia foetida etc.

A number of ayurvedic medicines have been prepared from above roots and herbs along with others for the treatment of arthritis & sciatica by Vaidyanath, Dabur, Jhandu & other companies. These medicines have been found to be very useful in controlling pain and inflammation.

2.4 HOMEOPATHY AND ARTHIRITIS

INTRODUCTION

Homeopathic medicines are made from animal, vegetable and mineral substances. These are prepared in such a way that they are nontoxic and do not show any side effects. The remedies are comparatively very cheap.

Homeopathic system of medicine is based on natural laws of healing. The most important fundamental law upon which homeopathy is based is 'Similia Simillibus curentur' i.e. like is cured by like. The law of similars enables a physician to prescribe a remedy based on characteristic symptoms.

A controlled process of successive dilutions, followed by succussions, called potentization prepares the homeopathic remedies. Lesser dilutions are called low potencies and higher dilutions are called high potencies. The process of potentization helps to use certain substances, which are otherwise inert like metals, charcoal etc.

There is a running quarrel amongst homeopaths between symptomatology and pathology. This dispute has no basic foundation because every symptom has its pathological significance. It is a different matter that we are not able to correlate every symptom to its pathological aspect. This is one of the reasons that most of the homeopaths prescribe on symptoms without insisting on pathology. However, pathological tests in many cases will definitely help in arriving at the correct medication.

The main principle of homeopathy is simillimum i.e. single remedy and minimum dose. Most of the homeopaths usually give one remedy at a time. The single remedy has been proved and tested on healthy people and hence it is very effective. Some homeopaths prescribe combination drugs. However, not many studies have been done as to what the effect of more than one medicine at a time would be or what is the interaction between the drugs.

Homeopaths believe that all parts of the body are interdependent and hence they treat the patient as a whole rather than concentrating on different organs separately. Homeopathy is truly holistic.

The symptoms of a particular drug can never be exhausted. It is very difficult to remember all the symptoms and even more difficult to apply this knowledge to the benefit of the patient. Each homeopath prescribes the drugs based on symptoms and pathology as per his own experience and genius. He takes into account certain aspects which may be completely ignored by others. The genius of the homeopath lies in extracting certain order in jumbled up symptoms of the drug and correlating it to the disease.

Hahneman maintained that the use of allopathic medicine is acceptable in acute diseases but in case of chronic diseases this method suppresses diseases causing more deep-rooted problems. However, even in acute diseases, it is possible to detect some symptoms which are characteristic of a particular person.

In conditions requiring surgery, homeopathic physicians use remedies before and after the operation. In certain deficiency states, conventional replacement therapy is a must and drugs like thyroxin, insulin, Vitamin $B_{12 \, etc}$. should be prescribed in normal doses. In some severe infections such as meningitis, tuberculosis etc, conventional antibiotics along with homeopathic drugs are found to be very useful.

In chronic diseases homeopathy sometimes achieves remarkable improvement when various forms of conventional therapies have failed. In some cases both types may complement each other. A patient with severe rheumatoid arthritis may require analgesic or anti-inflammatory drugs along with homeopathic remedies. Similarly an asthmatic patient may be given inhaler along with homeopathic drugs. With successful homeopathic prescribing, it is possible to stop administration of drugs, which cause undesirable side effects.

Chronic conditions often require regular and prolonged prescribing and do not expect rapid results in every case. However, in acute cases rapid response will occur with correct prescribing within hours or a day or two.

Sometimes in chronic cases, symptoms may be aggravated during the first week. It is due to the body's stimulus response to the remedy. The skin may be itchier, the joint more painful and even emotions stir up. This is a good sign and the response will follow soon.

Homeopathic remedies do not have long-term adverse effects but too many remedies given too frequently in high potency can cause profound disturbance and may cause difficulty for another prescriber. In such cases it is wise to stop all the remedies for few weeks.

In order to control arthritis, homeopathic medicines are required to control the following related conditions.

- Constipation and indigestion
- Obesity
- Diseases of bones
- Sciatica
- Osteo – arthritis &
- Rheumatoid arthritis

The different medicines and their characteristic symptoms are given in the following section. However, for the detailed study, works of Kent, Allen and Nash can be referred.

HOMEOPATHIC MEDICINES FOR CONSTIPATION

Different constitutional medicines for constipation are:

ALUMEN : There is an urge for stool all the time but there is no ability to expel the stool. Stool less frequent, drier and harder or in small pieces like sheep's dung. Intestines do not perform well. The patient suffers from cramps and colic pain.

ALUMINA : There is difficulty in passing stool, though stool is soft and sticky. There is no urging for stool until there is large accumulation. Condition aggravates after eating potato.

BRYONIA : A large, hard and dry stool which is passed with great difficulty. This is due to reduction in intestinal secretions and poor muscles. There is thirst for large drinks of cold water.

GRAPHITES : There is no urge to defecate for many days. Stool is large, knotty, united with mucus threads. There is pain during stool. Person is usually obese.

HYDRASTIS : Ten drops of mother tincture twice a day for few days is very useful to control constipation. When frequent use of purgatives causes constipation, this medicine is very useful.

MERCURIUS : Stool slimy, bloody, colic- pain during and after, cannot finish sensation. Moist tongue with intense thirst. Sweats day and night in many complains.

NATRUM MUR : Hard and crumbly stool, which causes rectal bleeding, soreness.

NUX VOMICA : Stool passes in small quan es and rectum does not clear fully. One gets relief after passing stool but gets the urge after sometime. Symptoms are heartburn, belching, bloating of stomach few hours after eating and even constipation. Person over indulges in tea, coffee, and tobacco.

SILICA : Due to insufficient expulsive power of rectum and sposmodic conditions, the stool starts out and goes back. There is soreness about the anus and oozing of mucus.

SULPHUR : Feces are hard, dark and dry. There is ineffective urging for stool with burning in anus. It is painful to pass stool owing to rectal fissures. Often treatment of constipation begins with Sulphur.

HOMEOPATHIC MEDICINES FOR INDIGESTION

ARGENTUM MET : Irresistible desire for sugar, gastric ailments with loud belching. Stool green with mucus like chopped spinach expelled with much sputtering. Withered and dried up person.

BRYONIA : Stomach is heavy after eating and sensitive to touch. Thirsty for large drinks of cold water but may vomit after taking a warm drink. You have bitter rising and may vomit bile and water. Least movement makes stomach worse.

CARBO VEG : Plainest food disagrees and causes gas and belching. Excessive flatulence, pressing upward in stomach and abdomen. Aversion to meat, milk & fatty foods. Craves for air.

CHAMOMILLA : Attack of indigestion follows a fit of anger and irritability. Stomach full of gas, cramping in stomach and bitter taste in mouth.

CHINA : Debility and other complains after loss of fluid or blood. Stomach feels full of gas that wouldn't come up or go down. Sweats with great thirst. Sweating during sleep and on getting covered.

LYCOPODIUM : Great flatulence with rumbling mostly intestinal with pressing downward. Increases from 4 to 8 P.M. after eating & in warm room. Great thirst after sweating.

NUX VOMICA : Hard diving zealous person, inclined to get excited and angry soon. Over indulges in food, coffee, liquor etc. Heartburn, belching and bloating of stomach a few hours after eating.

HOMEOPATHIC MEDICINES FOR OBESITY

The important remedies are:

CALCAREA CARB : Fair, fat, flabby and obese. Coldness general and local as if had a cold damp stockings. Afflictions from working in cold water. Sweats in general (night sweat and on exertion). Sweat on head, hands, feet etc. Can not walk far and go upstairs. Easily strained: Tardy development of bony tissues with lymphatic enlargement. Curvature of bones especially long bones. Skull very large. Feels a sort of inward coldness. Lower extremities cold. Longing for eggs especially in the children.

CROTON TIGLIUM : Sudden ejection of stool. Stools thin and yellow. There is excessive nausea but not much vomiting. Pain in intestine down to the anus. It is a stimulant of small intestine.

FUCUS VESICULOUS : It is a functional stimulant of thyroid

GRAPHITES : Especially adopted to persons inclined to obesity. Suited to women at the climacteric . Sad , despondent, hear better when in a noise. Sensation of cobwebs in the forehead. Stool knotty, large lump, united by mucous threads. Graphites cures complaints of many kind when there is a peculiar tendency to obesity and characteristic glutinous eruptions.

SPONGIA TOSTA : There is pain and sense of fullness in the region of heart. There is marked anxiety, fear of death and suffocation associated with palpitation and uneasiness in the region of heart. Spongia patient is worse from warm room and from heat. He wants to be cool. However, he is better from warm drink. Sore throat worse from eating sweet things. Thyroid gland swollen. At night there are suffocating spells with stinging in throat and soreness in abdomen. It is a functional stimulant of thyroid.

DISEASES OF BONES

ASAFOETIDA : Face looks puffed, bloated and dropsical. Inflammation of periosteum. Inflammation of cartilages. Person looks fat, flabby, purple. Numbness of scalp. Numbness after pain and after sleep. Hiccough like contraction of diaphragm with expulsion of wind. Wind and flatulence all press up.

CALCAREA CARB : Fat, flabby and obese. Produces deficient bones. Deficient teeth or no teeth. Feet cold and head warm, congestion in chest, anaemic, pale and waxy. Sweat of head with little exertion.

CALCAREA FLOUR : Indurated swelling of stony hardness in glands or ligament, bony infiltration in periosteum. This remedy has cured "Rice bodies" in cartilages. It can cure exostosis and indurate cervical gland.

CALCAREA PHOS : Night sweats. General bodily weakness. Numbness in many parts. Back pain worse in stormy weather and worse in the morning especially in the curvature in spine. Tearing, shooting pain in lower limbs. Non union of fracture bones. Polypi of nose, rectum and uterus. Enlarged glands of neck. Rachititis. Rheumatoid pains in joints and limb, worse from cold.

MEZEREUM : Pain in long bones especially tibia. Tearing pain in periosteum. Necrosis & carries etc.

PHOSPHORUS : Delicate, waxy and anaemic subjects. Small wounds bleed much. General dropsical condition. Bloating of hands and feet. Stiffness on beginning to move especially in the morning. Rheumatic stiffness in all limbs. Complains are worse with hot and warm applications. Soreness in places up and down the spine. Necrosis of lower jaw. Carries of other parts especially tibia.Craving for cold things, ice cream or cold water.He eats often or he faints.

SILICA : Silica patient is chilly. His symptoms are developed in cold damp weather. Symptoms come after bath. An offensive foot sweat which ceases after getting feet wet. Aversion to milk and diarrhea from milk. In childhood bones become soft and even necrose.

SYMPHYTUM : It is used for repair or reunion of bones.

THERIDION : Stitching and pain in left chest beneath the shoulder. Vertigo with nausea especially on closing the eyes. Very sensitive to sound which penetrates the entire body causing nausea and vertigo. In rachitis and caries, it goes to the root of the disease and destroys the cause.

SCIATIC PAIN

ACONITE : Complains from exposure to cold dry air. Increases in the evening, lying on left side, in warm room or warm covering. Decreases on uncovering. Dry hot skin and no sweat. Pain is attended with extreme restlessness & anxiety. Cannot bear to be touched.

AMMONIUM MURIATICUM : Sensation of coldness between the shoulders. Patient is worse when sitting, better when walking and fine when lying down.

ARSENIC ALBUM : Great restlessness and intense burning pain. Increases in cold air from cold things. Decreases by warm air, warm applications and by sweat. Patient cannot lie down, must sit and breathe. Pain, restlessness with reduced vitality, wants to move from place to place but not relieved. Important features of remedy are restlessness, burning, prostration and midnight aggravation.

CAUSTICUM : Pains of cramping and drawing nature. Contractions of ligaments. Drawing and tearing pain in legs, knees and feet. Contraction of muscles and tendons. Stiffness on rising from seat.

COLOCYNTHIS : Cramping pain in sciatic nerve from hip down to the thigh. Decreases by pressure and heat. Increases in the evening by anger and after eating.

GNAPHALIUM : Intense pain along the sciatic nerve alternating with numbness.

LYCOPODIUM : Sciatica pain starting from right and running to left. Burning sensation between the shoulders. Aggravation from 4 to 8 p.m.

MAGNESIA PHOS : Cramping pain everywhere. Increases by cold and cold application. Decreases by heat and pressure.

PHYTOLACCA DECANDRA : Pain travels down along the outside of the limb. Pain worse in wet weather and increases by motion. There is bruised and sore feeling. Phytolacca occupies a place mid way between Bryonia and Rhus tox.

RHUS TOX : Symptoms worse at night when resting but better, by movement, worse during cold and in the morning. Pain grows worse with change of weather. Improves by warmth but deteriorates in damp cold weather.

SPONDYLOSIS, ARTICULAR RHEUMATISM, SACROILIAC ARTHRITIS

BERBERIS VULGARIS : Main characteristic is bubbling sensation in the region of kidney. Pain in the region of kidney when stepping down stairs. Stiffness and lameness in the region of kidney. Increases in bed in the morning. Painful pressure in lumbar and renal region.

CALCAREA PHOS : Sleepy daytime and evening and sleepy in the morning. Stiffness in the morning. Aching in bones, worse from motion better during rest or from heat. Back pains worse in cold stormy weather and worse in the morning. Tearing, shooting pain in the morning. Weakness of muscles of the neck and long spine. Acts on the constitution.

CAUSTICUM : Pains of cramping and drawing nature. Drawing and tearing pain in legs, bones and feet. Contraction of muscles and tendons. Pains in loins when trying to get up. Painful rigidity of neck and dorsal muscles.

RHODODENDRON : Aggravation in wet stormy weather. Worse during rest but better during motion. However, it differs from Rhus tox in the sense that it is deeper seated and felt in periosteum as in teeth and bones of fore arm and tibia. Aggravation of symptoms before thunder storm i.e. rain and storm.

RHUS TOX : Lameness and stiffness on beginning to more and on getting up in the morning. Decreases by continued motion. Increases with damp cold weather, worse at night, resting. In general great nervousness.

OSTEO ARTHRITIS

ACID SULF: Weakness of spine : Stiffness of back when rising in the morning. Influences metabolism of cartilages.

ARGENTUM MET : Associated with degeneration of joints. It is full of tearing pain along the nerves, predominantly of lower extremities. Pain in cartilages and along the nerve and relieved by motion. Inflamed cartilages infiltrate and form into hard knots.

ARNICA : Whole body and extremities are cold but head feels hot. Arnica is useful in chronic cases of gout. There is soreness and tenderness of joints with great sensitiveness.

AURUM MET : Swelling of joints. Afflictions of cartilages and bones. Inflammation of periosteum. Thickening and induration of periosteum. Induration of glands and cartilages about the joints.

BRYONIA : Swelling of joints, great pain worse on touch or least motion. Joints red and stiff. Amelioration from pressure. Useful in second stage of inflammation of joints.

CAUSTICUM : Joint deformity with paralytic weakness and stiffness. Pain cramping and drawing in nature. Contractions of ligaments.

LEDUM PAL : Swelling is pale sometimes oedematous, increases at night, in the heat of bed. Cold water relieves. The joints become the seat of gout stones, which are painful.

RHEUMATOID ARTHRITIS

ACID SULF : Weakness of spine. Stiffness of back when rising in the morning. Influences metabolism of cartilages.

ACONITE : Complains from exposure to cold; increase in the evening, in warm room or warm covering; decrease on uncovering. Aconite is a pain remedy. Extreme restlessness and anxiety attend pain. Cannot bear the pain, nor bear to be touched. Trembling & tearing pain down the spine associated with sudden attack.

ACTAEA RECEMOSA : Muscular rheumatism, stiff neck, cannot move head. Rheumatism of belly muscles by preference.

ARGENTUM MET : Associated with degeneration of joints. It is full of tearing pains along the nerves, predominantly of lower extremities. Pain in cartilages, along the nerves and relieved by motion. Inflamed cartilage infiltrate and form into hard knots.

ARSENIC ALBUM : Restless, burning, prostration and midnight aggravation are some of the symptoms. Attacks the joints causing pale swelling and burning pain.

AURUM MET : Swelling of joints. Afflictions of cartilages and bones. Inflammation of periosteum, thickening and induration of periosteum. Induration of glands and cartilage about the joint.

BERBERIS VULGARIS : Pain with numbness in the region of kidney. Rheumatism of joint, pain which increases when stepping down.

BRYONIA : Dryness of mucous membranes, wants water in large quantities. Pain in joints, increases on movement. Joints swollen. Pain relieved by pressure on joint.

CACTUS GRANDIFLOROUS : Rheumatism of all joints beginning in upper extremities. Palpitation day and night worse when walking and lying on left side.

CALCAREA PHOS : Rheumatic pain in limbs in cold weather, worse from motion. Better during rest and from heat. Stiffness in morning. Aching in bones, gouty fingers and toes that become painful in cold weather.

CAUSTICUM : Pain cramping. Rheumatism of muscles and joints. Stiffness on rising from seat. Aggravation by cold.

CHAMOMILLA : Very irritable mood. Excessive uneasiness and anxiety. Violent rheumatic pains drive one out of bed at night.

CHINA : Complains after excessive loss of fluid. Blood from all outlets. Blood dark and clotted. General coldness. Sometimes convulsions. Cures inflammatory rheumatism.

DULCAMARA : Neck gets stiff after taking cold. Back painful. Tongue and jaw stiff. Tongue can even be paralyzed.

HEPAR SULF: Rheumatism when patient sweats day and night without relief.

KALI SULF : Rheumatic pain in joints moving from joint to joint. Chronic of Pulsatilla.

KALMIA LATIFOLIA : Useful in heart troubles of rheumatic origin. Rheumatism goes downward. Pain extends down to the left hand.

LAC CANINUM : Inflammatory symptoms moving from joint to joint when Pulsatilla fails.

LACTIC ACID : In addition to thirst, voracious hunger and profuse urine loaded with sugar, there is rheumatic pain in joints.

LEDUM PAL : Rheumatism begins in feet and travels upward. Swelling is pale sometimes oedematous. Increases at night in heat of bed. Rheumatic gout. The joints become seats of gout stones, which are painful. Cold water relieves the pain.

LILHIUM CARB : Chronic rheumatism connected with valvular heart disease. Rheumatic soreness in heart region. Pain in heart when bending.

MEDORRHINUM : Rheumatism of feet, ankles and soles. Pain worse in daytime.

MERCURIUS : Swollen flabby tongue. Gum swollen and bleeding. Breath offensive. Moist tongue with intense thirst. Pain in joints, increases after sweat. Worse at night in the warmth of bed.

NUX VOMICA : Zealous, over sensitive, easily excitable. Patient feels worse in the morning, after eating and in cold air. Body burning but person cannot uncover without feeling chilly.

PHYTOLACCA DECANDRA : In periosteal rheumatism. Pain worse in wet weather. Pain runs down the outer side of the limb as in sciatica. Increases with movement.

PULSATILLA : Mild gentle, yielding disposition. Muscles soft and flabby. Dryness of mouth in the morning but no thirst. Swelling of joints, pain wandering from one joint to another. Increases in warm room and warm applications. Decreases in cold open air and cold food.

RHUS TOX : Pain with numbness, gets relief from movement. Relief by pressure.

STICTA PULMONARIA : Severe pain and pressure in forehead. Sticta promptly cures rheumatism of knee joint.

SULPHUR : Burning everywhere, general, local and especially in feet. Redness of orifices as if full of blood. Bryonia and Sulphur complement each other.

VALERIANA : Pain worse when standing and letting the foot on the floor.

2.5 ACUPRESSURE SYSTEM OF MEDICINE

INTRODUCTION

Acupressure is an art of treating diseases by applying pressure on specific points of the body of the patient with the help of thumb or other blunt objects.

Identification of Acupressure points is end product of millions of detailed observations. It has been demonstrated that common painful diseases cause painful points in well-defined anatomical locations. Pressure on these points alleviates pains.

Acupressure points were subsequently grouped into a system of channels, which run into the body. At places these channels rise to the surface of the body while at others they go deeper into the body leading to the organ.

Channels create a network in body and are paired. One of the channels has yin characteristic while the other has yang. The numbering of points from yin channel starts from feet towards head since yin energy is supposed to come from

S. No.	Name of channel and type	Function
1.	Kidney–Yin Organ	Governs birth, growth and reproduction.
2.	Bladder–Yang Organ	Excrete fluids.
3.	Liver–Yin organ	Stores blood at rest and releases it during activity. Controls physiological functions and ability to plan.
4.	Gall–bladder–Yang organ	Stores and empties bile received from liver
5.,6.	Heart and heart protector. Yin organ.	Helps blood circulation. Influences clear thinking and long term memory.
7.	Tripple heater–Yang organ	Distributes and regulates warmth.

8.	Small intestine–Yang Organ	Receives food from stomach and separates nutrients from the waste.
9.	Spleen–Yin Organ	Transforms nutrients to help production of blood. Aids memory and concentration.
10.	Stomach–Yang organ	Churns and digests food.
11.	Lungs–Yin organ	Combine energy with air and spread it throughout the body via channel and blood vessels.
12.	Large intestine–Yang organ	Receives food material from small intestine, absorbs fluids and excretes stool.

earth. The points on yang channels are numbered from the head downward since yang energy comes from sun. The details of channels are given in table.

There are twelve channels each linked to the function of a particular organ. Besides, there are two more channels called *governor vessel* and *conception vessel*. *Conception vessel* is on the mid line of spine starting from half way between coccyx and anus passing through middle of top of head half way between ears to middle of furrow between upper lip and the nose. All channels except governing vessel and conception vessel are symmetric about mid line i.e. same points are located in same places on the opposite side of the body. Transversely the body has been divided in three parts. They are on the upper part of toes and fingers of hands and feet. The second part contains points of parts of body

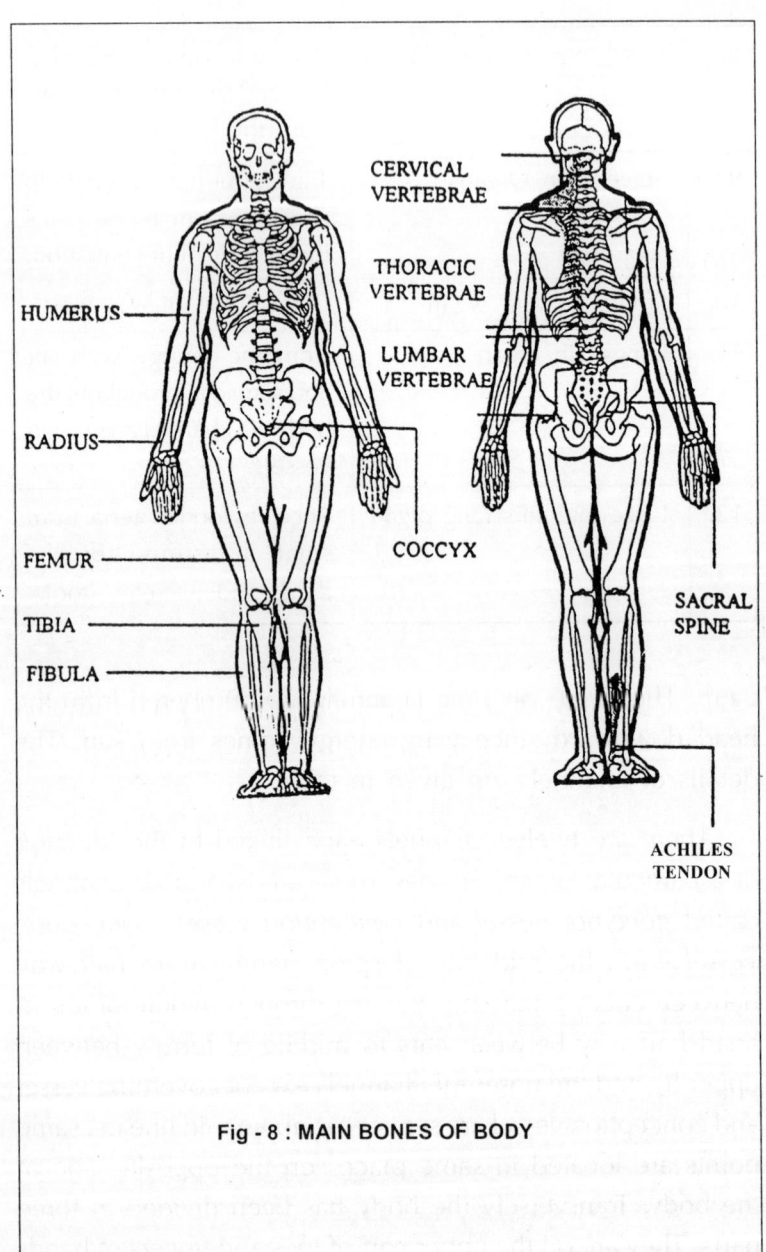

Fig - 8 : MAIN BONES OF BODY

below neck and above the diaphragm. The third part contains points corresponding to parts of body below diaphragm. (Fig.9)

There are approximately 900 points all over the body. Pressure is applied on these points to cure different ailments or to create an anesthetic effect.

Most of the organs and endocrine glands are to the left or right side of body so the corresponding points are on right or left palms and soles. The gall bladder, liver and appendix are to the right of body and their corresponding points are only on right palm and sole. Similarly, heart and spleen are on left side of body and their corresponding points are on the left palm and sole.

Further the body is divided into two parts i.e. front and back. For lower lumbago, sciatic nerves, nervous system and hips, pressure should be applied to the back of palms and soles. However, for other organs and endocrine glands, the pressure is to be applied on the front of the palms or soles.

ACUPRESSURE AND DISEASES

Diseases result when body is weak and unable to resist the onslaught of pathogens. These pathogens allow diseases to be grouped according to their broad symptoms.

The muscular aches that occur in association with viral infection would be classed as invasion by wind. People often complain that they catch chill when they get wet or their neck is stiff after sleeping in draught. If one has fever, heat is one of the causative factors involved in the disease process. Heat must be used to treat it. Other factors that cause disease are worry, anxiety, eating contaminated food etc.

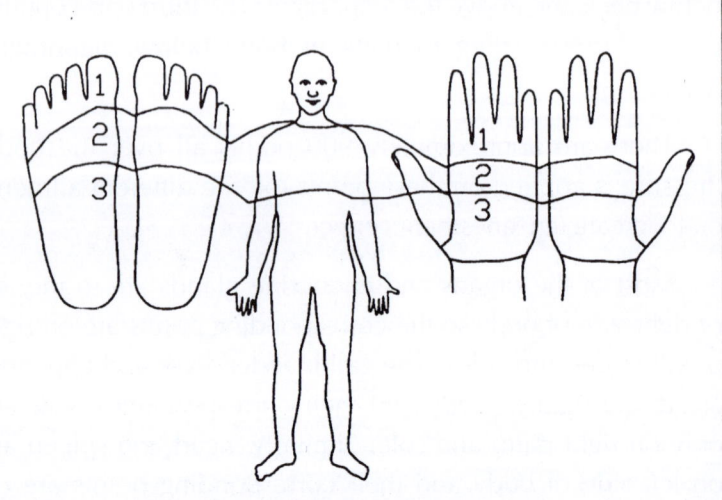

Fig - 9 : TRANSVERSE SECTION OF BODY

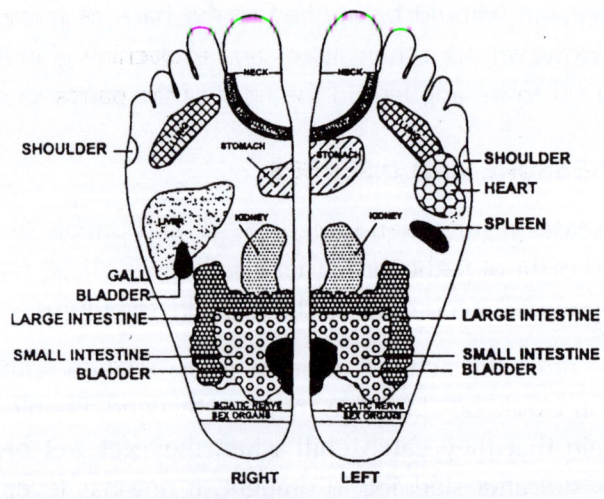

Fig - 10 : ACUPRESSURE POINTS OF DIFFERENT ORGANS IN FEET

The simplest and most obvious application of acupressure technique is in acute and chronic pain. The points can be selected by locating the most tender trigger zones.

However, in many diseases and in case of pain, associated symptoms may be present. This might include anxiety, depression or abdominal symptoms and indigestion, which are sometimes produced by analgesic and for anti-inflammatory agents. In such cases, it may be difficult to select points purely based on patient's localization of pain. In diseases like asthma, points selected cannot be based on tender point localization. It requires knowledge of traditional Chinese medicine. The biggest problem for any acupressurist is to define a set of points, which are clinically, most effective.

There are a large number of exceptionally well documented observations which lead us to infer that acupressure is having a fundamental effect on physiological functions which apparently modify the transmission and perception of pain.

In case there is no response to acupressure after first three sessions, it is doubtful whether any response will occur. Besides, the patient may sometimes experience a worsening of symptoms due to acupressure. It is a good sign and will last for a day or two followed by improvement. In case of musculoskeletal pain, acupressure does emerge as a consistently better analgesic therapy compared to other treatment.

DIFFERENT DISORDERS OF JOINTS, BONES AND MUSCLES

Before treating any of the above disorders, it is necessary to see that the central nervous system passing through the spinal cord is in order.

The central nervous system consists of brain, sciatic nerve and large number of nerves coming out of sciatic nerve which spread all over the body. Whenever there is any disturbance in the spinal cord, the part of the body connected to that point is affected.

The spinal cord passes through the vertebral column. The length of vertebral column of an adult is 60-70 cm. There are 33 vertebrae, which are connected to vertebral column. Out of these 33 vertebrae, 24 are separate and mobile bones while nine are fused. In the neck, there are seven cervical vertebrae, in upper back there are 12 thoracic vertebrae and in lower back there are 5 lumbar vertebrae. In the pelvic region there are five fused sacral vertebrae and four fused coccygeal vertebrae.

Thirty-one pairs of nerves are connected to spinal cord. These nerves are connected with different parts of the body. The connection between the different organs of the body and different parts of vertebral column is given below:

7 Cervical vertebrae

No. of vertebrae	Connecting organ of body
1.	Skull, mouth, brain, ears and blood circulation to head.
2.	Eyes, forehead, tongue, optic nerve and sinus.
3.	Cheek, teeth, outer ear, bones of face.
4.	Mouth, lips, nose, Eustachian tube.
5.	Vocal cord, pharynx, glands in the neck.
6.	Tonsils, shoulders and muscles of neck.
7.	Elbow, thyroid gland, shoulder & bursa.

12 Thoracic vertebrae

No. of vertebrae	Connecting organ of body
1.	Forearm and hand, trachea and oesophagous.
2.	Heart valves and coronary vessels.
3.	Chest, lungs, breasts, bronchial tubes.
4.	Gall bladder and its duct.
5.	Liver, solar plexus
6.	Stomach
7.	Duodenum, pancreas
8.	Spleen, diaphragm
9.	Adrenal glands
10.	Kidneys
11.	Ureters and kidneys
12.	Small intestine, fallopian tube and circulation

5. Lumbar vertebrae

No. of vertebrae	Connecting organ of body
1.	Large intestine
2.	Abdomen, appendix, thigh
3.	Sex organs, bladder, knee
4.	Sciatic nerve, lowback muscles and prostate
5.	Leg, ankles, feet.

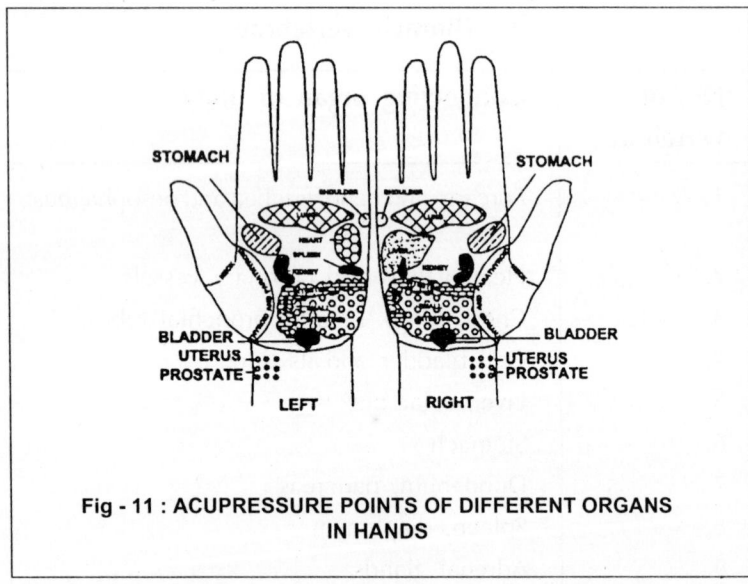

Fig - 11 : ACUPRESSURE POINTS OF DIFFERENT ORGANS IN HANDS

Sacral – 5 – fused sacral vertebrae - Hips

Coccyx – 4 Fused Coccygeal vertebrae - Rectum, anus

Accupressure therapy entails application of pressure to the corresponding points of vertebral column in addition to the point of that organ. It is possible that the main cause of disease is in the vertebral column. For this purpose one should check the vertebral column as follows:

Lie down on your stomach with arms straight on sides. You will observe two round depressions on both sides of spine in the lumbar region. In case these depressions are not visible, the problem of the system is mainly due to spinal cord. In case the depression is on the left side only, the problem is connected with spinal cord and in the right side. Similarly if depression is on right side only, the problem is in the left side of spinal cord. Run two fingers from first cord

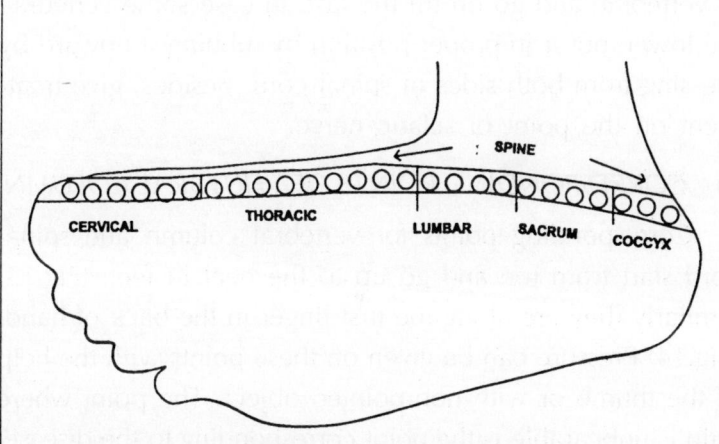

Fig - 13 : POINTS OF VERTEBRAL COLUMN IN FOOT

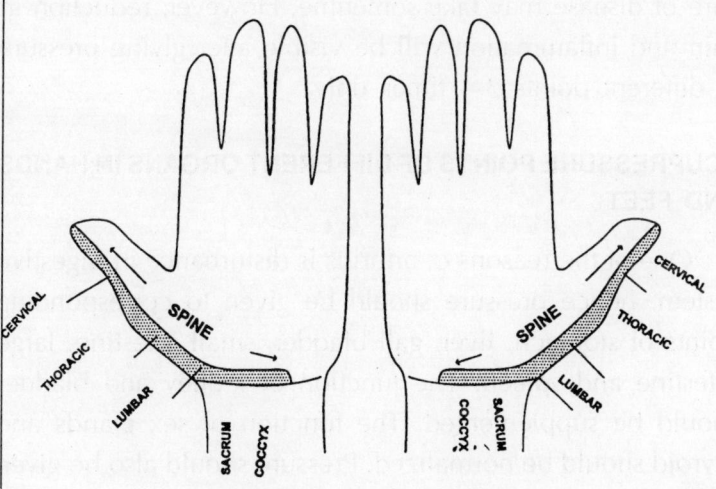

Fig - 14 : POINTS OF VERTEBRAL COLUMN HANDS

of vertebrae and go on till the last. In case some vertebrae are lower, put it in proper position by rubbing it upward by pressing from both sides of spinal cord. Besides, give treatment on the point of sciatic nerve.

- **CORRESPONDING POINTS OF VERTEBRAL COLUMN:**

Corresponding points for vertebral column and spinal cord start from toe and go up to the heel in feet. (Fig.13) Similarly they are along the first finger in the back of hand. (Fig.14) Pressure can be given on these points with the help of the thumb or with non-pointed object. The point where pain is unbearable is the point corresponding to the disease.

We shall now discuss different techniques of acupressure to cure different disorders.

Depending on severity of disease, it is possible that the cure of disease may take sometime. However, reduction in pain and inflammation will be visible after giving pressure to different points 3-4 times only.

ACUPRESSURE POINTS OF DIFFERENT ORGANS IN HANDS AND FEET

One of the reasons of arthritis is disturbance in digestive system, hence pressure should be given to corresponding points of stomach, liver, gall bladder, small intestine, large intestine and spleen. The function of kidney and bladder should be supplemented. The function of sex glands and thyroid should be normalized. Pressure should also be given to points of nervous system. (Fig.10 & 11)

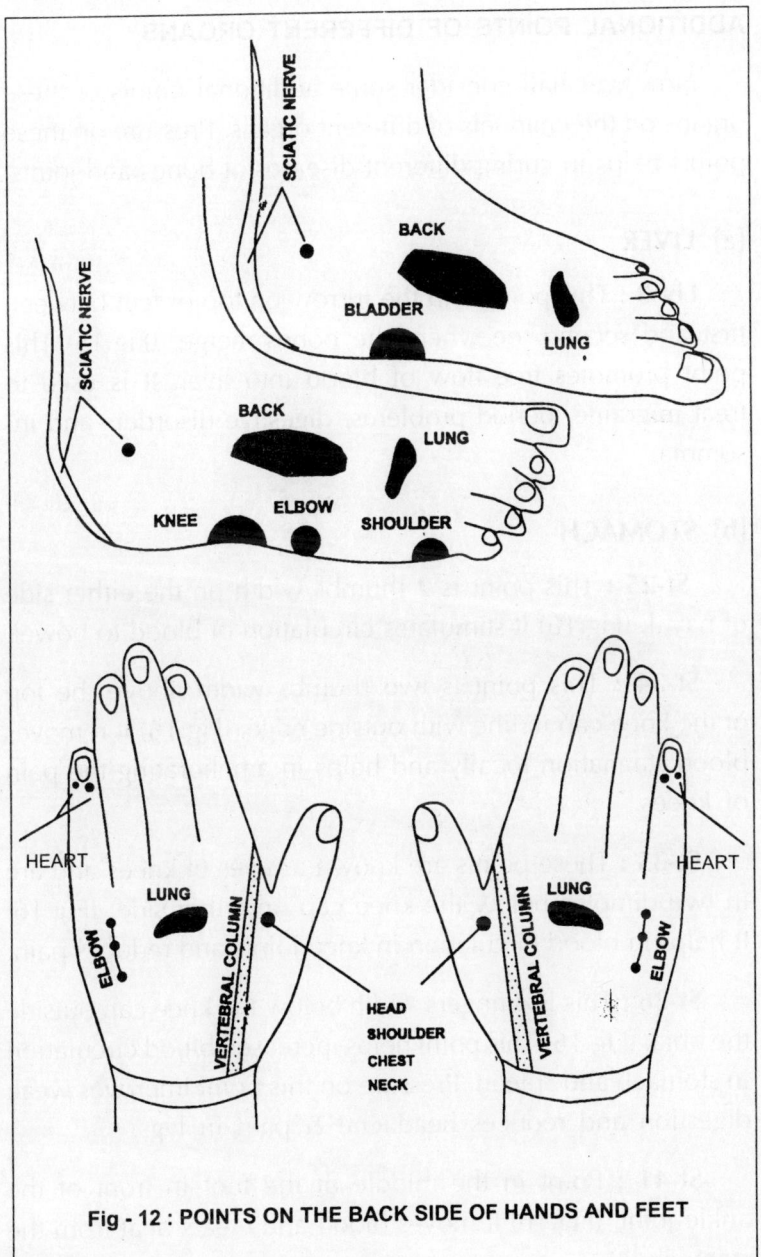

Fig - 12 : POINTS ON THE BACK SIDE OF HANDS AND FEET

ADDITIONAL POINTS OF DIFFERENT ORGANS

Now we shall consider some additional points of these organs on the channels of different organs. Pressure on these points helps in curing different diseases of bones and joints.

[a] LIVER

Liv-3 : This point is in the furrow on top of feet between first and second toe where the bones merge. (Fig.15) This point promotes free flow of blood into liver. It is used to treat migraine, period problems, digestive disorders and insomnia.

[b] STOMACH

St-25 : This point is 2 thumbs width on the either side of naval. (Fig.16) It stimulates circulation of blood to bowel.

St-34 : This point is two thumbs width above the top of the knee cap in line with outside edge. (Fig.16) It removes blood stagnation locally and helps in ameliorating the pain of knees.

St-35 : These points are known as eyes of knees and are in two dimples below the knee cap on either side. (Fig.16) It helps in blood circulation in knee joints and reduces pain.

St-36 : This is 4 fingers width below the knee cap outside the tibia. (Fig.16) This point helps increased blood circulation in stomach and spleen. Pressure on this point improves weak digestion and reduces headache & pain in legs.

St-41 : Point in the middle of the foot in front of the ankle joint. (Fig.16) It moves blood and clears heat from the stomach.

St-43 : This point is in furrow between the 2nd and 3rd toe where the bones merge . (Fig.16) It cools down stomach and helps in reducing acidity.

St-44 : This point is in web at the base of second and third toe on the top of foot. (Fig.16) It removes fullness and heat from stomach.

[c] KIDNEY

K-3 : This point is between inside ankle bone and Achilles tendon. (Fig.15) Pressure on this point strengthens kidney.

K-6 : This point is one thumb below the inside ankle bone at the junction of bone and muscle. (Fig.15) Pressure on this point nourishes kidney and eliminates heat.

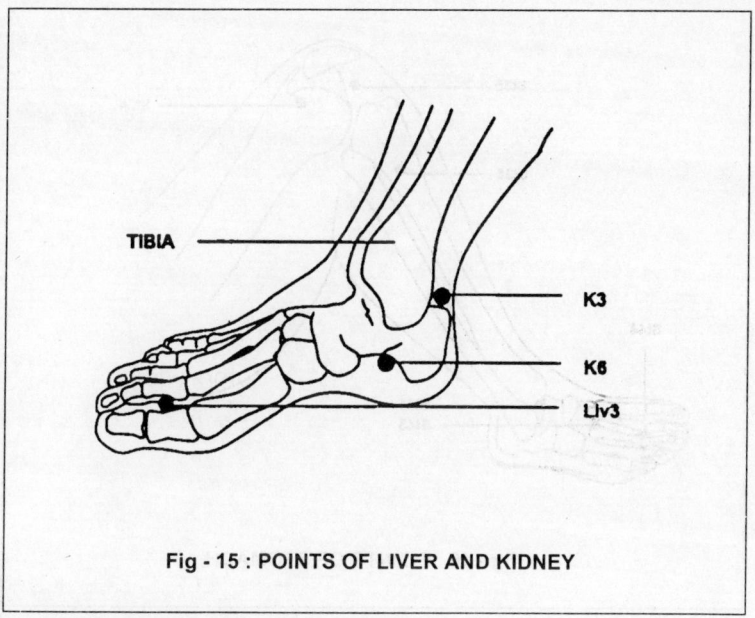

Fig - 15 : POINTS OF LIVER AND KIDNEY

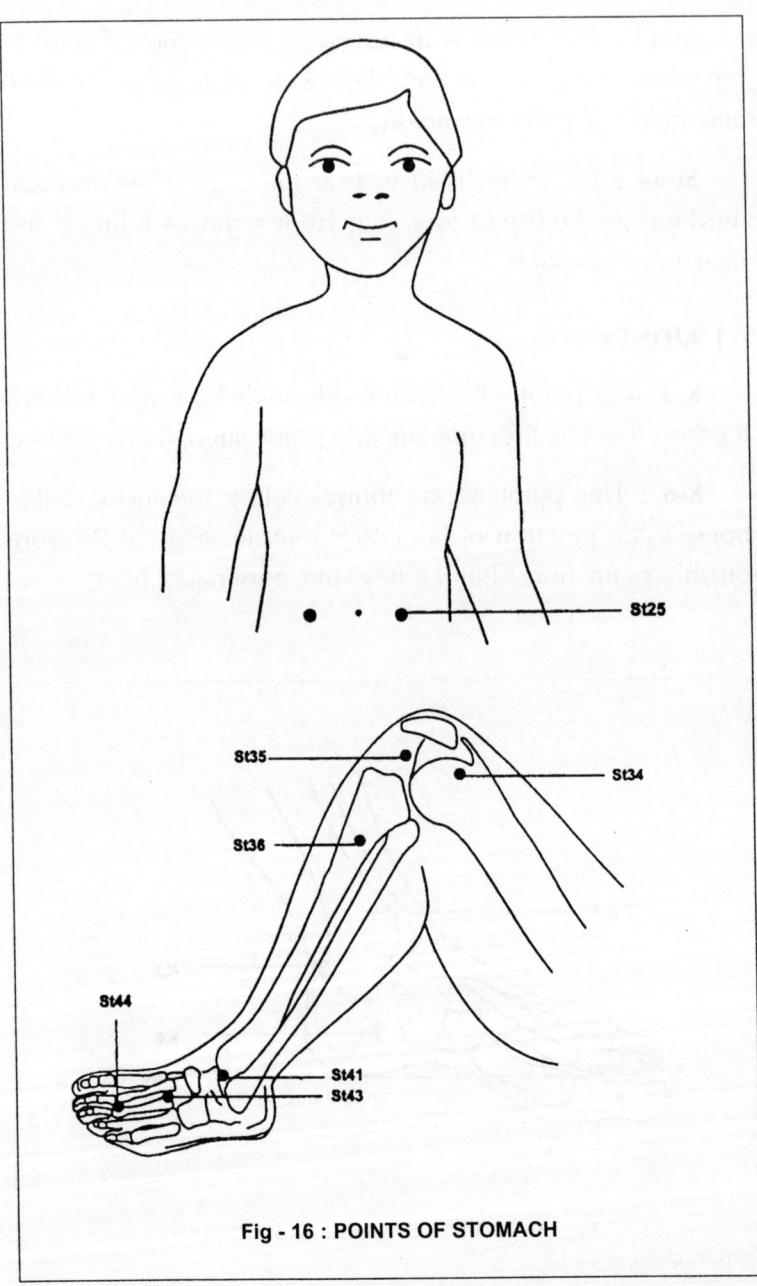

Fig - 16 : POINTS OF STOMACH

[d] SPLEEN

SP-4 : This point is on the inside arch of foot just under the base of big toe. (Fig.17) It calms down the stomach.

SP-6 : This point is 4 fingers width above the inside ankle bone just behind tibia. (Fig.17) It stimulates circulation and production of blood and eliminates dampness. It is good for poor digestion and anemia.

SP-9 : The point is on the inside of leg below the knee joint in depression between tibia and calf muscle. (Fig.17) It helps in blood circulation and in removing dampness and heat from knee joint.

SP-10 : This point is two thumbs width above the top of knee cap and two thumbs width towards the inside of thigh. (Fig.17) It helps in blood circulation in the knee joint.

[e] SMALL INTESTINE

SI-3 : The point is on the back of the hand between the bone and muscle just before knuckle of little finger. (Fig.18) It improves blood circulation in hand and wrist.

SI-5 : The point is in hollow on the little finger side of wrist joint. (Fig.18) This point clears heat from small intestine channel. It improves blood circulation in wrist.

SI-12 : The point is in the middle of muscle above, the ridge of shoulder blade midway between cervical spine and the tip of shoulder. (Fig.18) Pressure on this point increases blood circulation in neck and shoulder.

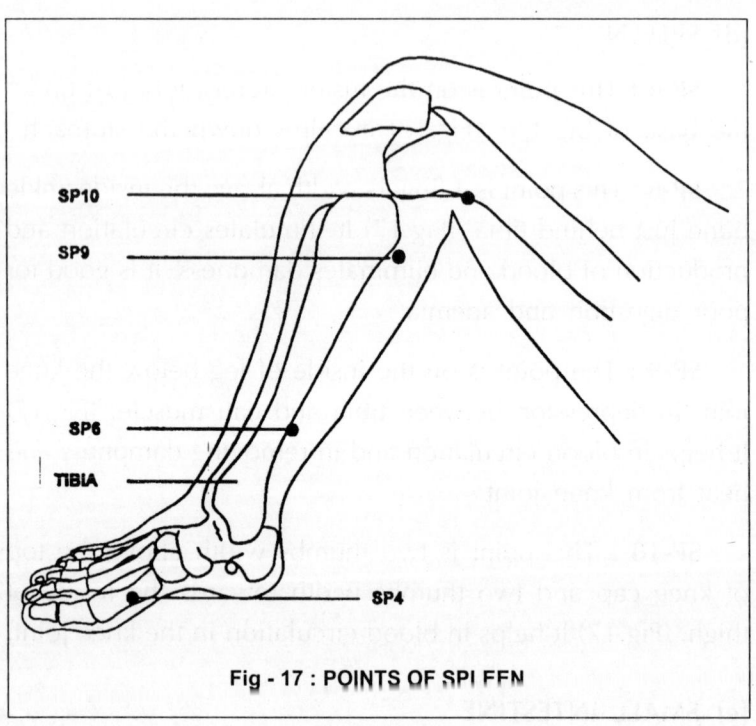

Fig - 17 : POINTS OF SPLEEN

[f] LARGE INTESTINE

LI-4 : It is located in the web between the thumb and the index finger on the back of hand. (Fig.18) It assists in bowel movement and clears wind. It is useful in reducing and curing headache, toothache, sinusitis, cold and pain in the upper body.

LI-5 : It is in the hollow at the base of the thumb on the side of the wrist joint. (Fig.18) It improves blood circulation in the wrist and clears heat from the large intestine.

LI-10 : It is two thumbs width below the crease on the outer side of the elbow in line with the middle of the back

Treatment of Arthritis

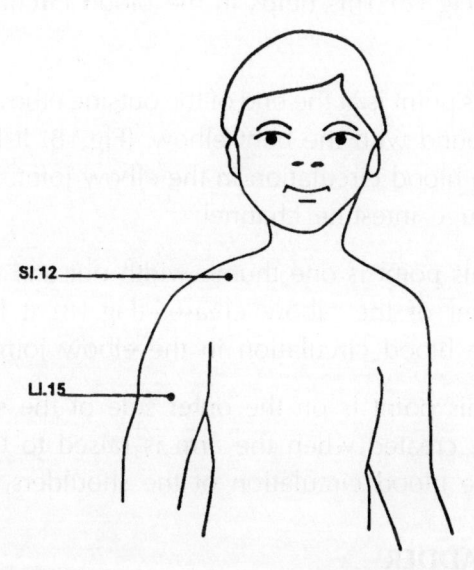

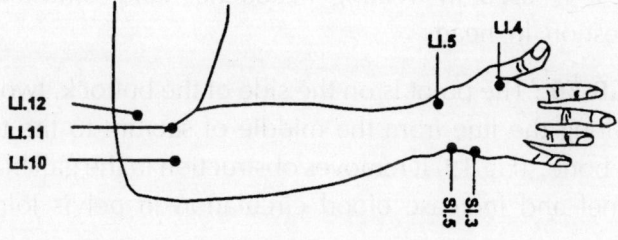

Fig - 18 : POINTS OF SMALL INTESTINE AND LARGE INTESTINE

of the wrist. (Fig.18) This helps in the blood circulation of the arm.

LI-11 : This point is at the end of the outside elbow crease and can be found with the bent elbow. (Fig.18) It helps in improving the blood circulation in the elbow joint. It clears heat in the large intestine channel.

LI-12 : This point is one thumb width out and up from the outer point of the elbow crease. (Fig.18) It helps in improving the blood circulation in the elbow joint.

LI-15 : This point is on the outer side of the shoulder in the dimple created when the arm is raised to the side. It helps in the blood circulation of the shoulders.

[g] GALL BLADDER

GB-20 : This point is found at the base of the skull in the hollow between the front and the back neck muscles behind the ears. (Fig.19) This point clears wind and calms liver. It is used in treating headache, cold, sinusitis and congestion in head.

GB-30 : The point is on the side of the buttock, two third out along the line from the middle of sacrum to the top of thigh bone. (Fig.19) It removes obstruction in the gall bladder channel and increase blood circulation in pelvis Joint.

GB-31 : This point is on the outside of the thigh 3-4 inch in width above the outside crease of the knee joint. (Fig.19) It removes obstruction in gall bladder channel and relaxes tendons.

GB-34 : This point is on the depression on the outer side of the lower leg below the knee joint in front and below

Treatment of Arthritis

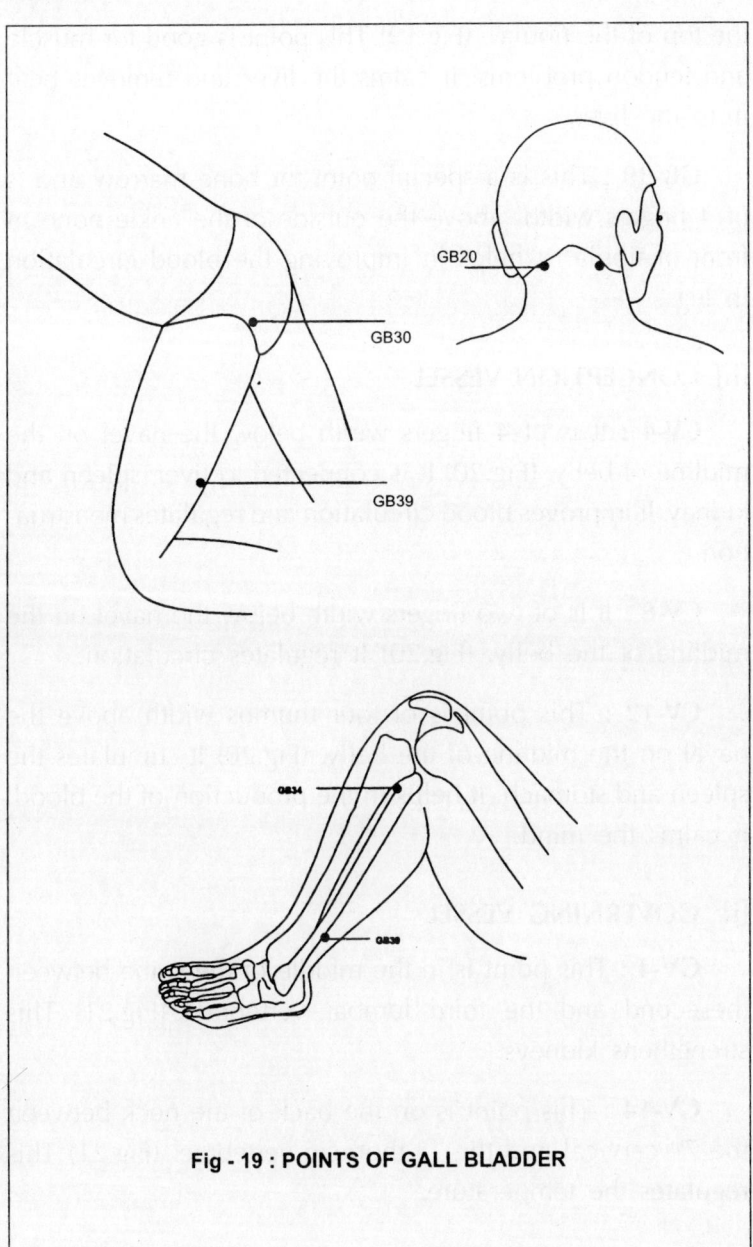

Fig - 19 : POINTS OF GALL BLADDER

the top of the fibula. (Fig.19) This point is good for muscle and tendon problems. It calms the liver and removes heat from the liver.

GB-39 : This is a special point for bone marrow and is of 4 fingers width, above the outside of the ankle bone in front of fibula. It helps in improving the blood circulation in legs.

[h] CONCEPTION VESSEL

CV-4 : It is of 4 fingers width below the navel on the midline of belly. (Fig.20) It is connected to liver, spleen and kidney. It improves blood circulation and regulates menstruation.

CV-6 : It is of two fingers width below the navel on the midline of the belly. (Fig.20) It regulates circulation.

CV-12 : This point is of four thumbs width above the naval on the midline of the belly. (Fig.20) It stimulates the spleen and stomach. It helps in the production of the blood. It calms the mind.

[i] GOVERNING VESSEL

GV-4 : This point is in the middle of the spine between thesecond and the third lumbar vertebrae. (Fig.21) This strengthens kidneys.

GV-14 : This point is on the back of the neck between the 7th cervical and the 1st thoracic vertebrae. (Fig.21) This regulates the temperature.

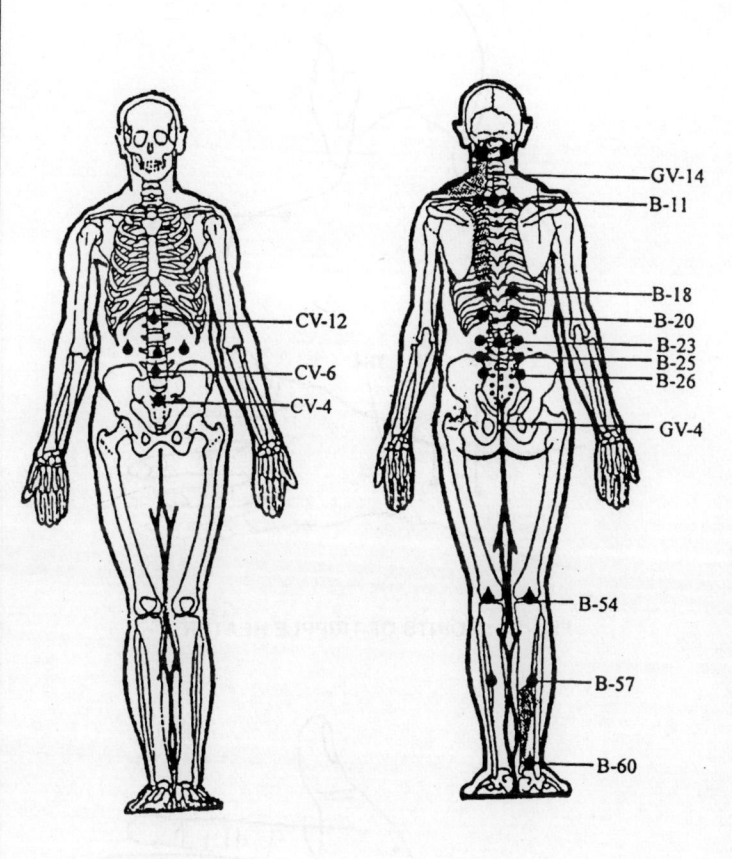

Fig - 20 : POINTS OF BLADDER, GOVERNING VESSEL AND CONCEPTUAL VESSEL

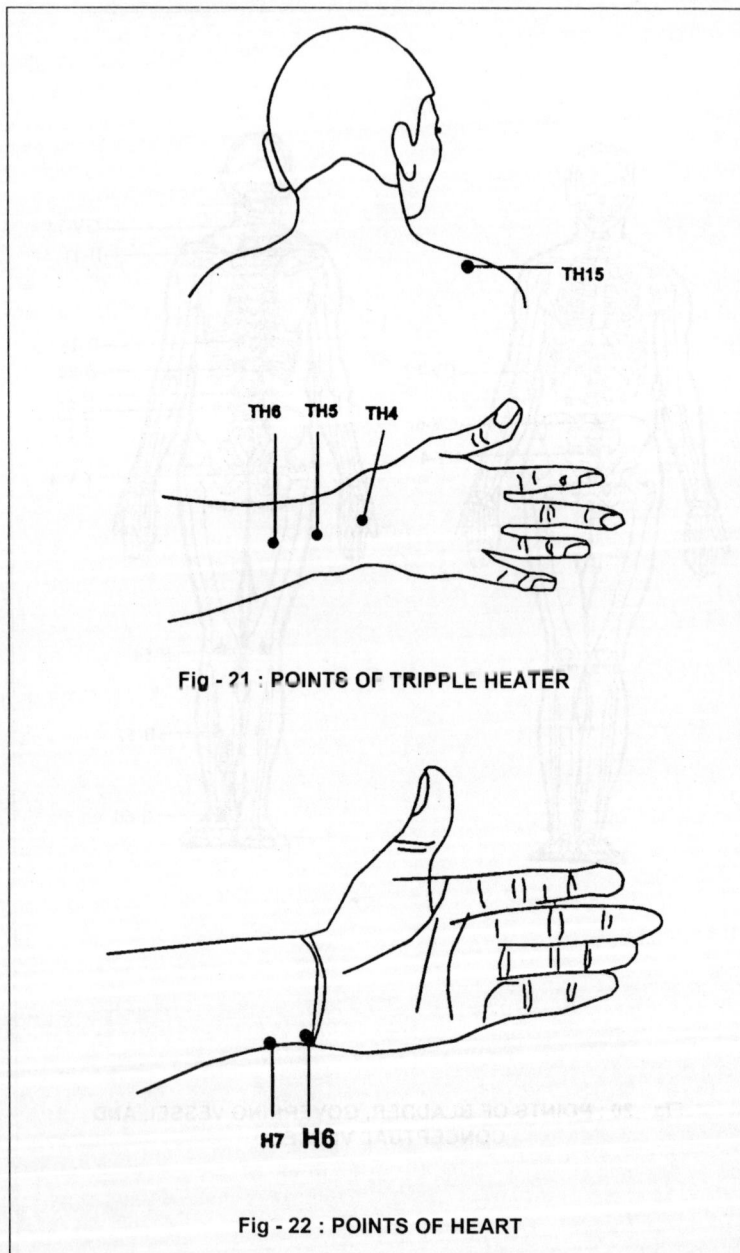

Fig - 21 : POINTS OF TRIPPLE HEATER

Fig - 22 : POINTS OF HEART

[j] TRIPPLE HEATER

TH-4 : This point is in the middle of the wrist joint on the back of the hand. (Fig.21) It helps in the blood circulation and relaxes the tendons.

TH-5 : This point in two-thumbs width, above the wrist crease in the the middle of the back of the forearm. (Fig.21) It relaxes tendons.

TH-6 : This point is of four fingers width above the wrist on the back of the forearm. (Fig.21) It helps in blood circulation.

TH-15 : This point is above the ridge of the shoulder blade just down from the highest point of the trapezius neck muscle. (Fig.21) It is midway between cervical spine and tip of shoulder. It helps blood circulation in neck muscles.

[k] BLADDER

B-11 : This point is the about one inch width on the either side of the spine between the 1st and 2nd thoracic vertebrae. (Fig.20) It clears wind and is useful in ailments of the trachea, hands and arms.

B-18 : It is about an inch on the either side of the spine level with 9th and 10th thoracic vertebrae. (Fig.20) This point regulates spleen and adrenal glands and helps in blood circulation.

B-20 : This point is about an inch on either side of the spine level with 11th and 12th thoracic vertebrae. (Fig.20) It regulates kidney and small intestine.

B-23 : This point is about one inch on the either side of spine level with 2nd and 3rd lumbar vertebrae. This helps in the blood circulation in the breasts, lungs, trachea etc.

B-25 : This point is about an inch on the either side of the spine level with 4th and 5th lumbar vertebrae. (Fig.20) It is useful in ailments of sciatica, prostate, hands, feet and ankle.

B-26 : This point is about an inch on the either side of spine level with 5th lumbar and 1st sacral vertebrae. It helps in the blood circulation and strengthens ligaments which stabilize lumbar and sacral spine.

B-54 : This point is in the middle of the crease on the back of the knee. (Fig.20) It helps in the blood circulation in the lower leg and removes dampness.

B-57 : This point is in the middle of the back of the calf where muscles and tendons meet. (Fig.20) The point helps in blood circulation in this area.

B-60 : This point is on the outside of the ankle halfway between the ankle bone and the Achilles tendon. (Fig.20) This reduces pain in the back and clears heat.

[I] HEART

H6 : This point is of half a thumb width from the wrist crease on the forearm on the little finger side of the palm. (Fig.22) It moves blood circulation and heat affecting the heart. It helps in stopping hot flushes and night sweats and calms the mind.

H7 : The point is on little finger side of the wrist crease. (Fig.22) It calms mind and improves blood circulation in the heart and the chest.

DISORDERS OF NECK AND SHOULDER JOINTS

Neck and shoulder joints are shallow and are supported by ligaments and tendons. They allow wide variety and range of movements.

Any injury or distortion in this part causes a number of ailments, some of them are:
- Cervical spondylosis
- Cervical spondylitis
- Inflammation of bursa in the armpit
- Stiff neck
- Vertigo-illusion of revolving motion either of oneself or one's surroundings
- Shoulder pain or frozen shoulder
- Pain and numbness in hands and fingers.

Contrary to popular belief, common use of cervical collar by spondylitis patient is not recommended. In severe cases of spondylitis, collar can be used when one is under taking long journeys etc. Similarly, traction in every case of cervical spondylitis may aggravate the disease.

In all the above disorders pressure on the following points is recommended.

i. The internal and external part of the thumb of the right hand and leg is connected to the right side of the neck. Similarly internal and external part of thethumb of the left hand and foot is connected to the left outer side of the neck. The upper part of the thumb is connected to the upper part of the neck while the lower part is connected to the lower part of the neck. The pressure is to be given to the corresponding point of the thumb for curing ailment.

ii. Pressure should be given to the point where the neck and the skull meet i.e. the starting point of the vertebral column. Pressure should be given in for 3-5 seconds three times.

iii. Pressure to be given at the base of the skull in a hollow between the front and back neck muscles behind the bony prominence. (GB-20)

iv. Corresponding point of neck and shoulder are also there in the palm of hands and feet and pressure should be given on them.

v. In the middle of the muscle above the ridge of the shoulder blade midway between cervical spine and the tip of the shoulder (SI-12)

vi. Find this point on the outside of the shoulder in the dimple created when the arm is raised to the side. (LI –15)

vii. Point is located in the web between the thumb and the index finger on the back of the hand. (LI-4)

DISORDERS OF THE ELBOW JOINT

The elbow is a shallow joint, which is supported by overlapping of ligaments and tendons. Most injuries damage these ligaments and tendons. Pain in the elbow can be due to cervical spondylosis and over use of hands resulting in pulling of the muscles of the hand.

In order to control pain in elbow (tennis elbow), in addition to giving pressure on the points for control of cervical spondylosis, the pressure should be given on the following points.

  i. Point one thumb width up from the outer point of the elbow crease. It is between the muscle and the upper arm bone. (LI-12)
  ii. Point two-thumb width above the wrist crease in the middle of the back of the forearm. (TH-5)
  iii. It is at the end of the outside crease of the elbow. (LI – 11)
  iv. Located in the web between , the thumb and the index finger on the back of the hand. (LI-4)
  v. It is two- thumb below the crease on the outer side of the elbow. (Point–LI-10)
  vi. It is in the depression of the outer side of the lower leg below the top of the fibula. It is a point for the muscle and tendons. (Point GB –34)

DISORDERS OF HAND AND WRIST JOINTS

Hand and wrist joints are strong and allow a wide range of movement. When one falls, he automatically put hands to save himself and this leads to wrist injuries. There may be pain or swelling around the ligament or a bone fracture. Pain may also be due to some disturbance in the nervous system.

In addition to the general points of the joints, the following specific points should be pressed.

  i. Points in the web between the thumb and index finger on the back of the hand. (LI-4)

ii. Point on the back of the hand between the bone and the muscle just before the knuckle of the little finger. (SI-3)

iii. In the hollow at the base of the thumb on the side of the wrist joint (Point no.LI-5)

iv. In the hollow on the little finger side of the wrist joint (SI-5)

v. In case of numbness of hand and fingers, pressure on the point on the wrist crease and half a thumb width on the wrist crease on the little finger side of the palm. (H-6 & H-7)

DISORDERS OF PELVIS JOINT AND LUMBAR REGION

The pelvis joint is a ball and socket joint. It allows maximum stability but only a narrow range of movements. The lumbar spine and pelvis consist of large bones with ligaments and muscular support. Wear and tear and stiffness are very common. It may be caused by spondylosis or arthritis, due to bad lifting habits and wrong posture.

In addition to general points, the pressure on the following points is very helpful.

i. Points on the side of the buttock, two third out along the line from the middle of the sacrum to the top of the thighbone. (GB-30)

ii. Points about one inch on either side of the spine at the level with the 5th lumbar and first sacral vertebrae. (B-26)

iii. Points about one inch on the either side of the spine between 2nd & 3rd lumbar vertebrae. (B-23)

iv. Point in the middle of the crease on the back of the knee (B-54)

DISORDERS OF THE ANKLE JOINT

They are designed to take all your weight and still be flexible. It is a strong joint but is easily twisted. It may cause ligament damage with pain and swelling. In order to cure the ankle, the pressure should be applied on the following points.

  i. Point between inside anklebone and Achilles tendon. (K-3)
  ii. Point in the middle of the foot in front of the ankle joint. (St-41)
  iii. Point on the outside of the ankle halfway between the ankle bone and Achilles tendon. (B-60)
  iv. Point in the depression on the outerside of the lower leg below the knee joint. It is in front of and below the top of fibula. (GB-34)

DISORDERS OF KNEE JOINT

Knees take lot of weight of our body. They are very stable. Injury in knee may result in damage to cartilages and ligaments. The pain in knee also results from athritis. In order to cure the knees the pressure on following points should be given.

  i. Corresponding points in front and back of hands and feet.
  ii. Points in the middle of crease on back of the knee. It improves circulation in the lower leg. (B-57)

iii. There are two dimples below the kneecap, called eyes of the knee. (St-35)

iv. Point two thumbs above the knee cap and two thumb points towards inside of the thigh. (SP-10)

v. Point two thumbs width above the top of the knee cap inline with its outside edge. (St-34)

vi. Point on the inside of the leg below the knee joint in the depression the between tibia and the calf muscle. (St-34)

vii. Point 4 finger width below the tip of the knee cap outside the tibia. (St-36)

SCIATIC PAIN

Sciatic nerve is an important nerve of our nervous system. It starts from the spinal cord at the 4th and 5th lumbar vertebrae. It passes through the back of the thigh. Before reaching the knee, it is divided into two parts. It reaches near the ankle after passing through the internal and back portion of the leg.

The pain in the leg associated with the disease is mainly due to injury in the inter vertebral disc. The pain starts from hips, travels down the back of the thigh and the outside of the leg and extends to as far as the ankle and the foot. At times loss of feeling and numbness is found. When sciatica is present, there will be nerve root pressure in the lumbar region at the bottom of the spine. It may also result in back pain.

There are a number of reasons for nerve pain. The important one's are:

- Malformation of bones in lumbar region.
- Prolapsed inter vertebral disc.
- Diseases of urinary bladder, uterus and ovaries.
- Lifting heavy weights or injury.

For the treatment of sciatica pressure should be given to the points corresponding to:

i. Kidneys and bladder

ii. Points in hands and feet corresponding to lumbar and sacral vertebrae.

iii. Points relating to sex glands

iv. Points on the outside of ankle, halfway between outside ankle bone and Achilles tendon. (B-60)

v. Point on the side of the buttock, two third out along the line from middle of the sacrum to the top of the the thigh (GB-30)

vi. Point on the outside of the thigh about 3-4 inches above the outside crease of the joint (GB-31)

vii. In the depression on the outside of the leg below knee joint in front of and below the top of fibula (GB-34)

viii. Point 4 finger width above the outside ankle bone in front of the fibula (GB-39)

ix. Point in the middle of crease on the back of knee. (B-54)

x. Point in the middle of the back or calf where muscle and tendon meet. (B-57)

xi. Points about one inch on either side of the spine at the level of the 5th lumbar and 1st sacral vertebrae. (B-6)

xii. Points about one inch on either side of the spine at the level of the 2nd & 3rd lumbar vertebra. (B-23)

DISORDERS OF BACKBONE

Backache may be due to back weakness or due to injury. Poor posture and lack of exercise contribute to the problem. It may also be due to spondylosis and spondylitis. In order to control backache, the following precautions should be taken:

i. When you sit on a chair or sofa, your back should be straight and knee comparatively higher than hips.

ii. You should not be overweight. In standing position, the body should be straight.

iii. Do not do any work while bending. In case you have to work sit, on your feet and do the work.

iv. In case you lift anything, lift equal weight from both the hands.

v. Keep your back straight while doing house work or driving a vehicle etc.

vi. Sleep on hard bed and use light cotton couch. Incase of pain in neck use thin cotton pillow.

vii. After lying down, one should not get up straight but should get up side ways putting weight of body on arms.

The lumbar region can also become painful if you do not drink enough water. In this case kidneys will not function properly and will result in toxicity causing pain.

In order to cure back pain give pressure on the following points.

- Points about one inch on either side of the spine at the level of 2nd and 3rd lumbar vertebrae (B-23)
- Points about one inch on both sides of the spine at the level of 4th and 5th lumbar vertebrae.(B-25)
- Points on the spine between 2nd and 3rd lumbar vertebrae. (GV-4)

Acupressure points for controlling constipation and indigestion are discussed as under:

CONSTIPATION

In Constipation pressure on following points will help:

i. Keep one hand on other on the right side of belly and produce wave like motion from your hands. The rhythm should be slow and graceful.
ii. Point in the middle of chin, hard pressure should be given to this point.
iii. Point located in the web between thumb and index finger on the back of the hand. It assists bowels and clears wind. (LI-4)
iv. Point about an inch on either side of spine level with 4th and 5th lumbar vertebrae. (B-25)
v. Point about one inch on either side of spine level with 9th and 10th thoracic vertebrae (B-18)
vi. Point of 2 thumb width on the either side of the navel (St-25)
vii. Point in the middle of wrist joint on the back of hand (Th-4)
viii. Points of liver and stomach in hands and feet

INDIGESTION

Pressure on following points will help.

i. Points of liver and stomach in hand and feet.

ii. Point four thumb width above the naval on the midline of the belly. (CV-12)

iii. Point two thumb width on either side of the naval. (St-25)

iv. Points four finger width below the knee cap on the outside of tibia. (St-36)

2.6 YOGA AND MOBILITY OF JOINTS

INTRODUCTION

In case of arthritis there is severe inflammation in the joints. In order to allow maximum healing to take place naturally, it is advisable to take rest for one to two weeks. It is also recommended to take medicines to control severe pain and inflammation. Continuous pain for a long time usually reduces the amount of exercise we take and the muscle of the body becomes weak. Slowly even the efficiency of the heart and lung will also suffer.

It is not only necessary to plan exercise after rest but it is important to do exercises of right kind and proper duration. Wrong exercises and doing them too much will be very harmful. It will produce exhaustion and increase the intensity of pain. It will further frustrate the patient and reduce his will power to start it again. When the patient starts exercises in the beginning, he is normally enraged and feels further frustration as during exercise he feels pain but slowly as the muscles are strengthened the pain is reduced and he gets confidence. The exercise works as a painkiller.

The mobility of a joint is key to managing pain, resuming normal activity and finally to rehabilitation. Exercise stimulates the production of endorphins in the bloodstream and increases body's capacity to cope with pain.

In order to maintain the maximum mobility of joints, yogic exercises are the best. In this section we shall discuss about yogic exercises and their correlation with different arthritic disorders. During the practice of yogic exercises (asanas), there should not be rapid movement of the body and limbs and the breathing process should be normal. The mind should be at peace and should be withdrawn from all thoughts.

In yogic exercises, there is harmonious development of all muscles of body, internal organs and the nerves. The movements are gentle and rhythmic and there is minimum wastage of energy. In order to derive maximum , the following instructions should be followed.

i. Asanas should be done on empty stomach in the morning or 3 to 4 hours after taking food.
ii. Spread a folded blanket on the floor and practice yogic exercises.
iii. Before doing yogic exercise mind and body both should be relaxed.
iv. In the beginning, each asana should be practiced for a few seconds and gradually increase the duration. They should be done slowly.

v. Asanas should be practiced in well-ventilated room where there is free movement of clean air.

vi. In order to derive the maximum , be regular.

vii. Limitations mean asanas not to be done in those disorders & benefits mean asanas to be done in those disorders.

SOME IMPORTANT YOGIC EXERCISES.

YOGIC EXERCISES TO FACILITATE BOWEL MOVEMENT

Drink two glasses of lukewarm water in the morning with or without a little salt in it and do the following five exercises 8 – 10 times. (Fig.23) These exercises help in controlling constipation.

[a] TADASANA (Palm tree pose)

Stand straight with feet at a distance of 4-6" inches apart. Raise the arms above your head with palm upwards. See towards your hands. Now raise your heels and stretch the body fully in the upward direction. Balance your weight on fingers and slowly bring the heels to the ground. Repeat it 8 – 10 times.

Inhale while stretching upwards and exhale while coming down.

[b] TRIYAK TADASANA (Curved palm tree pose)

Stand as in Tadasana with heels raised and body stretched in the upward direction. Curve the body from the back first in the right direction and then in the left direction. Do this asana 10 times in each direction, and then stand on your feet.

In the beginning, it is difficult to balance the body weight on fingers. Hence, initially this exercise can be done by balancing the weight on the toes. Inhale while standing straight and exhale in curved movement.

[c] KATI CHAKRASANA (Circular movement of back)

Stand on feet with feet 2-3 feet apart. Spread the arms at the height of the shoulders on both sides. Upper part of the body is moved in a circular movement on right side such that left hand comes to right shoulder & right hand circles round the back. Repeat the exercise on the other side. Repeat it ten times.

[d] TRIYAK BHUJANGASANA (Curved cobra pose)

Lie on the ground with forehead touching the ground. Place your palms on the floor below the shoulders and spread the legs 2-3 feet apart. Press in the palms against the floor, inhale and slowly raise the upper part of body bending the vertebrae one by one until body from naval downward touches the floor. Curve the head and back in one direction and see the heel of other foot. Exhale in this position. Repeat this exercise in opposite direction.

Repeat the above exercise ten times in each direction.

[e] CROW MOVEMENT

Sit on your toes. Put your palms on the knees. Walk like a crow touching the knee on the ground on each step. Slowly do this exercise without tension for a minute.

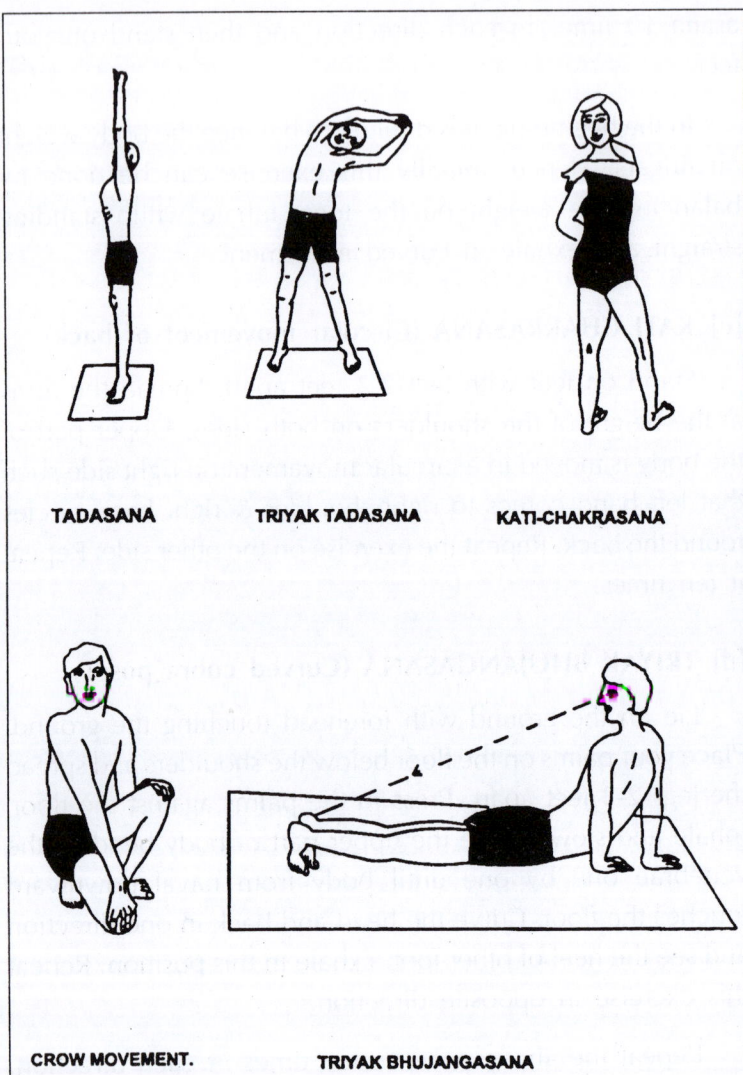

Fig - 23 : YOGIC EXCERCISE TO FACILITATE BOWEL MOVEMENT

YOGIC EXERCISES USEFUL IN GASTRIC TROUBLES

These exercises help in getting rid of gastric troubles. These are also helpful for persons suffering from indigestion and constipation. (Fig.24) The following exercises are very useful.

[a] ROTATING THE LEGS

Lie on your back with hands straight and on both sides of the body. Keeping your right leg straight, lift it above the ground and rotate it 5-10 times in clockwise direction and 5-10 times in anticlockwise direction. Repeat this exercise with left leg.

During this exercise the body along with the head should be touching the ground. After finishing this exercise take rest till breathing is normal.

[b] CYCLING

Lie on your back. Lift the right leg and rotate it like cycling. Do it 5-10 times in one direction and 5-10 times in opposite. Repeat it with left leg.

Practice cycling with both legs 5-10 times in one direction and 5-10 times in another.

During this exercise the body along with the head should be touching the ground. After every part of exercise take rest till breathing is normal.

[c] BENDING THE LEGS

Lie on your back. Bend your right leg and bring the thigh near the chest. Press the knee with your both hands and exhale. Now try to touch the nose to the knee raising the

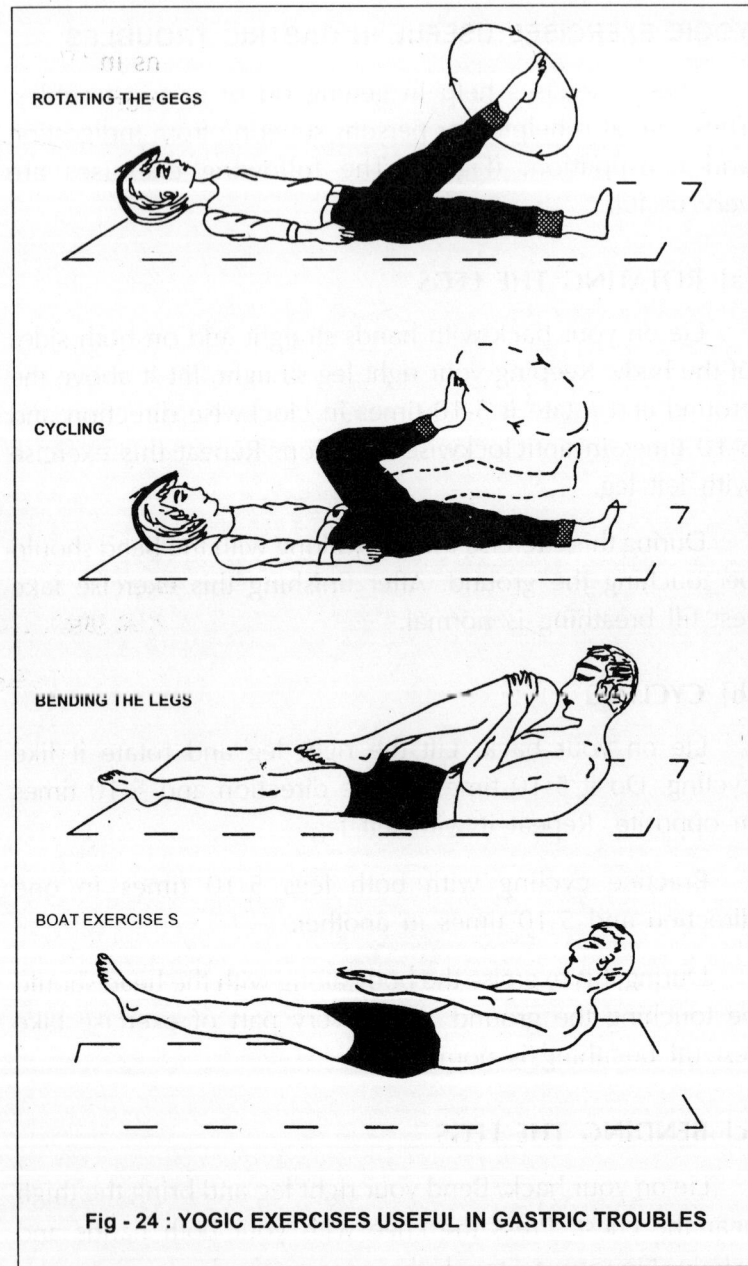

Fig - 24 : YOGIC EXERCISES USEFUL IN GASTRIC TROUBLES

head and the upper portion of the chest. Come to lying position inhaling slowly. Loosen the body. Repeat it 5-10 times. Repeat this exercise with the right leg.

Now bend both the legs and circle your arms around the knees. Repeat all actions as above. Breathing should be in harmony with the body movement.

[d] BOAT EXERCISE

Lie on your back with hands on both sides of the body and palm towards the ground. Inhaling, lift hands, arms, head and torso above the ground. Head should not be more than one foot above the ground. Arms should also be on the same height and fingers of feet should be straight, Keep yourself in this position as long as it is comfortable. Exhaling come to ground slowly. Relax. Repeat this exercise 5-10 times.

YOGIC EXERCISES FOR JOINTS

These exercises are very useful for joints and related body parts. (Fig.25A, 25B)

[a] CURLING THE FINGERS OF FEET

Sit with legs stretched and support your body with the hands by bending backward. Keep hands straight and do not curve the elbows. Curve the fingers of foot backward and forward. Repeat ten times.

[b] BENDING THE TOES (Feet stretch)

Sit in the position of exercise [a]. Bending from ankle move your toes away from yourself. Now bending at the ankle, bring the toes towards yourself as far as possible. Repeat it ten times.

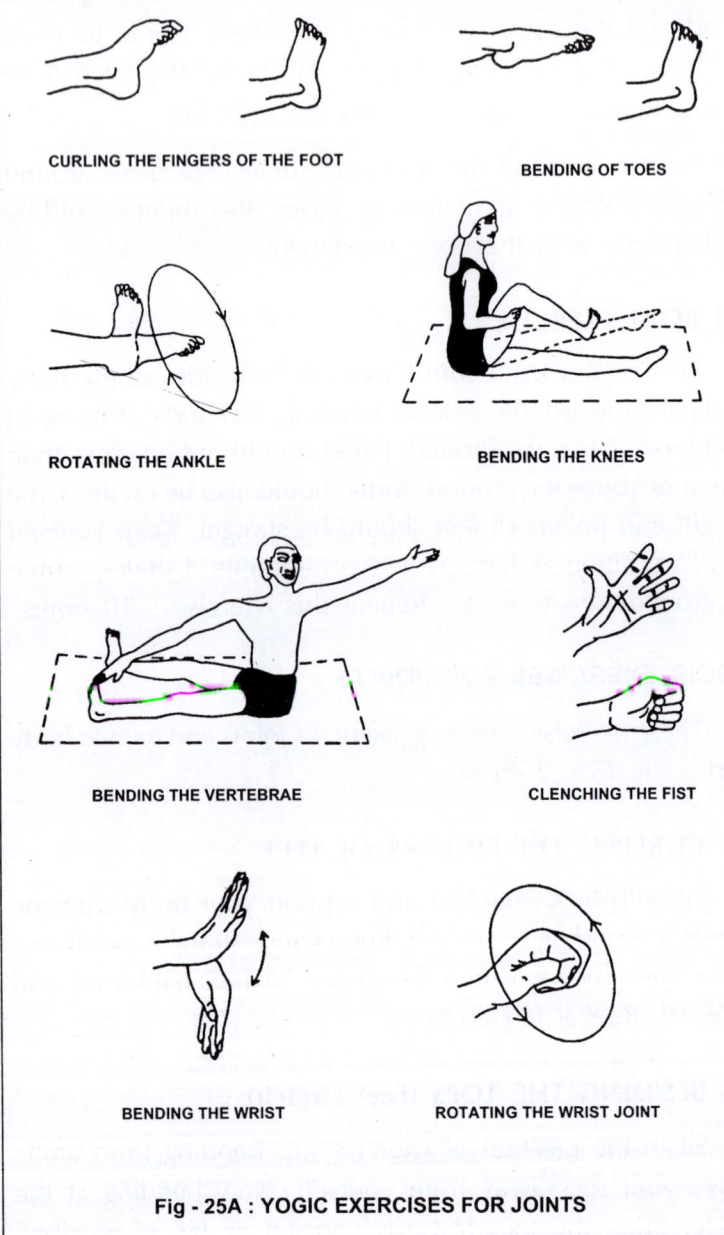

Fig - 25A : YOGIC EXERCISES FOR JOINTS

[c] ROTATING THE ANKLE

Sit in the position as in exercise [a]. Keep some distance between the feet. Keeping heels on the ground rotate each ankle first in clockwise and then in anticlockwise direction. Repeat ten times.

[d] BENDING THE KNEES

Sit straight with legs stretched. Bend the right knee and keep both hands tied behind the right thigh. Keeping hand below the right thigh near the knee, straighten the leg. The heel should not touch the floor. Bend the right leg from knee as far as possible and bring heel near right hip. Repeat it 10 times.

Similarly repeat this exercise with left leg.

[e] BENDING THE VERTEBRAE

Sit straight with legs fully stretched and 2-3 feet away from each other. Keeping hands straight bring the right hand near the toe of the left foot and stretch the left hand to the back side. Both arms should be in straight line. Bending the neck keep your sight towards the left arm.

Now do the exercise in opposite direction. This will constitute one frequency. Now repeat it 5-10 times.

[f] CLENCHING THE FIST

Stand straight. Spread the arms at shoulder level parallel to the floor. Spreading fingers of both hands, produce tension in it. Keeping the toe inside, clench the fist. Again spread the fingers and produce tension. Repeat it 10 times.

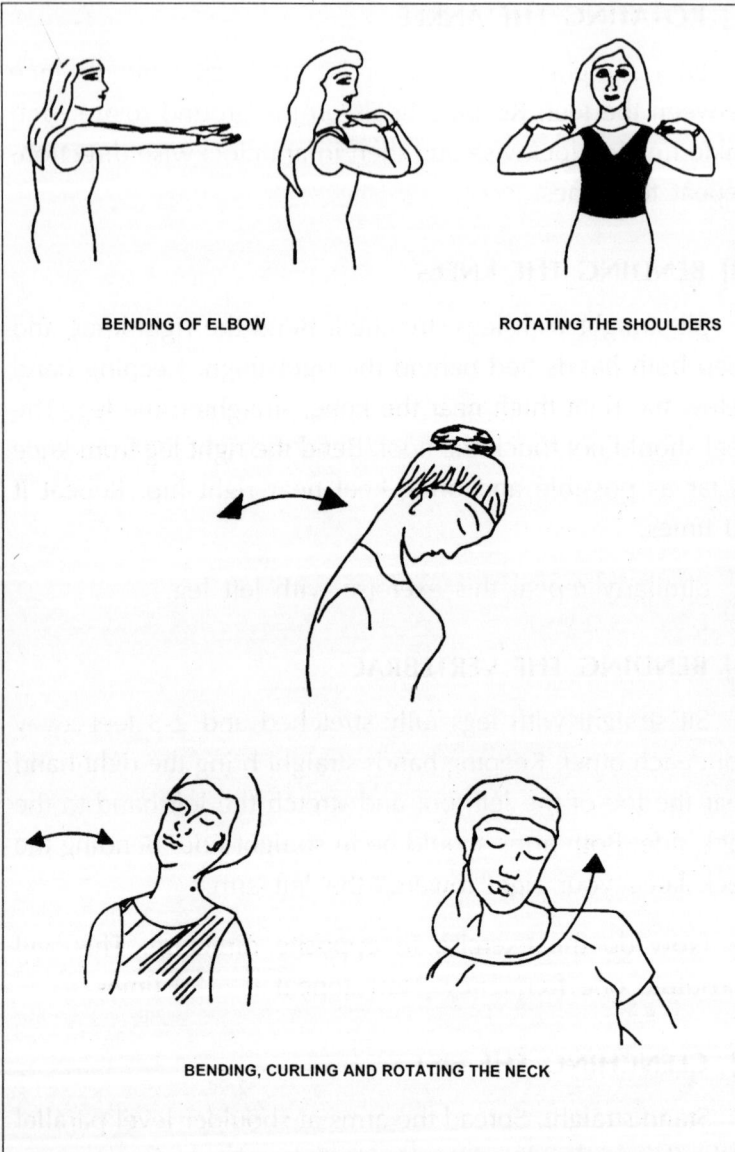

Fig - 25B : YOGIC EXERCISES FOR JOINTS

[g] BENDING THE WRIST

Take positions as in exercise [f] with fist open. Bend the palm from the wrist in the upward direction keeping fingers straight. Now bend the palm from the wrist in the downward direction. Repeat it 10 times.

[h] ROTATING THE WRIST JOINT

Take position as in exercise.[f]. Clench the fist of the right hand. First rotate in clockwise direction and then in anti clockwise direction. It should be repeated ten times. Repeat it with left hand. Exercise should also be repeated with both hands simultaneously.

[i] BENDING OF ELBOW

Take positions as in exercise [f] with the fist open and the palm in the upper side. Bending the arms from elbows, touch the fingers to the shoulder. Then straighten the arms at shoulder level. Repeat it 10 times.

Straighten the arms to the side and repeat the exercise 10 times.

[j] ROTATING THE SHOULDERS

Take position as in exercise [i]. Keeping the fingers at the shoulders, rotate the shoulders first in clockwise direction and then in anti-clockwise direction. Try to make the circle as large as possible and let the elbows touch each other in front of the chest. Repeat it 10 times.

[k] BENDING, CURLING AND ROTATING THE NECK

Sit down with legs straight and hands on both sides of the thighs on the floor.

- Bend the head forward and backward 10 times.
- Keeping face straight bend the head sideways on right and on left 10 times each
- Rotate the head in as big a circle as possible first in clockwise direction and then in anti-clockwise direction. Repeat 10 times in each direction.

VAJRASANA AND RELATED ASANAS

These exercises are very easy but very effective. These exercises are very useful in controlling the nervous system. They control sex glands and are also useful in digestion of food. Different exercises in this group are as follows. (Fig.26A, 26B)

[a] VAJRASANA (ADAMANT POSE)

Sit kneeling, knees and toes together and heels apart. Sit between the heels. Body erect, hand on thighs and eyes closed. Breathing normal. Keep the spine and neck straight.

The body acquires stability in this pose. This posture strengthens the waist & muscles of legs, tones up the nervous system, and helps in digestion of food. This is also a good asana for meditation and prayer.

LIMITATIONS : This exercise is not suitable for persons with gross osteo-arthritis of knees and other painful conditions of knees and ankles.

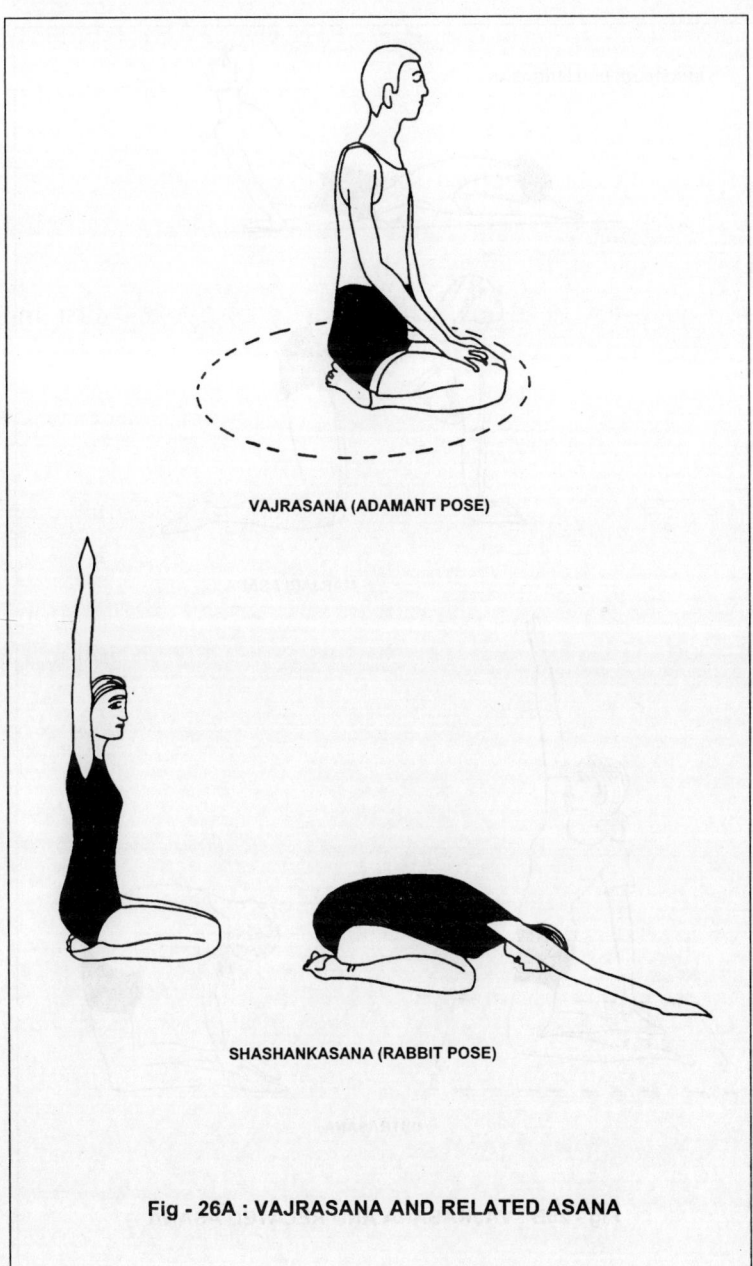

Fig - 26A : VAJRASANA AND RELATED ASANA

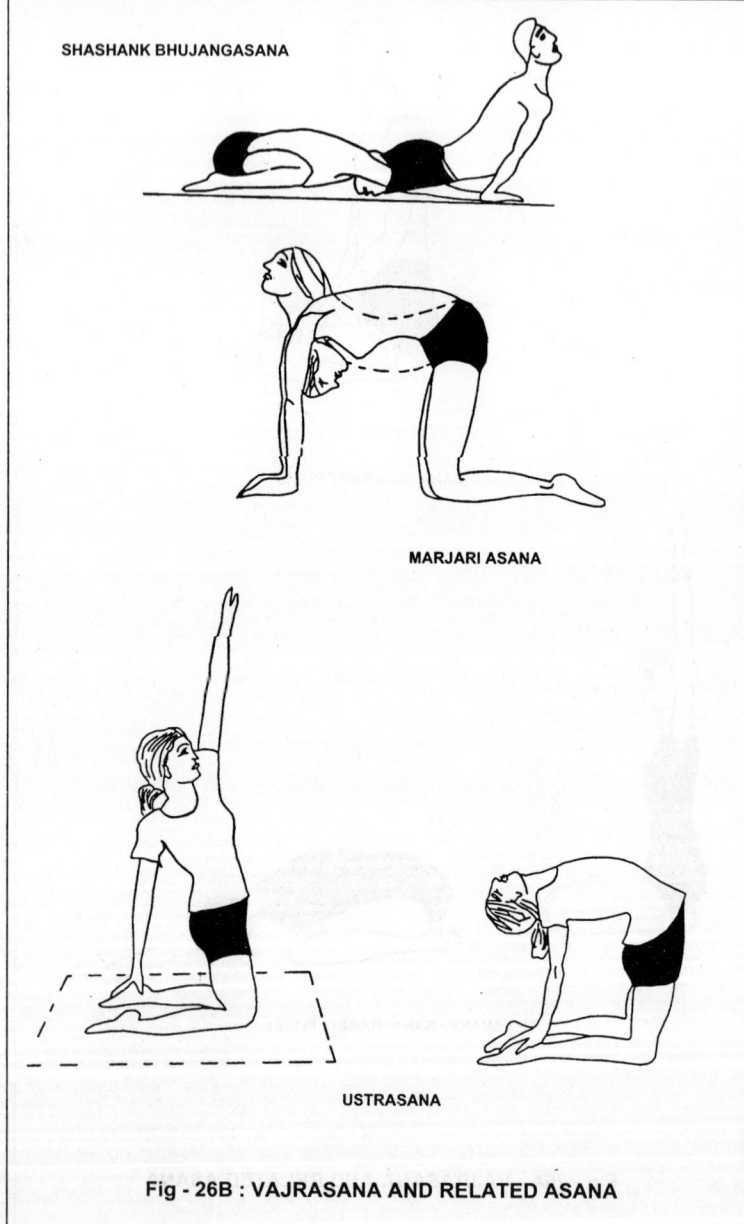

Fig - 26B : VAJRASANA AND RELATED ASANA

[b] SHASHANKASANA (RABBIT POSE)

Sit in vajrasana with hands on knees. While inhaling lift hands above head. Keeping hands in line with torso, touch the floor with forehead and exhale in the process. For few seconds keep the breath out. Now inhaling slowly take the hands above the head in line of torso. While exhaling come to the initial position. Repeat it 10 times.

A variation of this exercise can be done by taking the hands to the back and holding wrist of the right hand with the left hand and vice versa.

BENEFITS : This asana exercises sciatic nerve and regulates adrenal gland. It also helps in proper development of breasts.

LIMITATIONS : This exercise is not recommended for persons with gross osteo-arthritis of knees and other painful conditions of knees and ankles.

[c] MARJARI ASANA (CAT POSE)

Sit in vajrasana. Kneel with hands straight just below the shoulders. Keep the spine in straight line with floor. Breathe in, hollow your back and raise your head. Breathe out, arch your back and bring the head towards the chest. Repeat it 10 times.

BENEFITS : This exercise is useful in gynaecological troubles. It makes neck, shoulder & spine flexible.

[d] SHASHANK BHUJANGASANA (RABBIT AND COBRAPOSE)

Come in marjari asana and keep hands 45 cm apart. Without displacing hands take the chest forward touching the floor till it is in straight line with the arms. Touch the stomach on the floor and take the chest further forward till it is bow shaped. Now bend the head backward (snake pose). Now slowly take the back upwards, and taking the head and the entire body backward come to the postion of shashankasana (rabbit pose). Stay in this position for few seconds and return to marjari asana (cat pose)

Breathe normally in cat pose. Breathe in while going to snake pose and breathe out while returning to the rabbit pose.

BENEFITS : This exercise is useful in disorders of stomach, liver, sciatica and gynaecological troubles.

[e] USTRASANA (CAMEL POSE)

There are two variations of this exercise.

- Sit in vajrasana. Keep distance between the knees. Stand on knees. Turn the torso to your right and bending backward hold the heel of the left leg with your right hand. Raise your left hand over your head straight and look towards it. Now allow the weight of your upper body on the heel of the left leg. Repeat it in opposite direction.

  Breathe in while standing on knees. Breathe out while turning. Again breathe in while bringing torso in the middle.

- Come in position (a) of Ustrasana. Bend the neck and torso as far as possible in the backward direction. Come in the original position.

Breathe in while standing on knees. Breathe out while bending backward.

BENEFITS : This exercise is very useful in digestion, gynaecological troubles and back pain.

LIMITATIONS : This exercise is not recommended for persons with gross osteo-arthritis of knees and other painful conditions of knees and ankles.

EXERCISES OF BENDING BACKWARD

These exercises are very good in diseases of back and spine. They are also very useful for the nervous system which passes through the spine. The most important asanas of this group are Bhujangasana (Cobra pose), Shalbhasana (Locust pose) and Dhanurasana (Bow pose). (Fig.27)

[a] BHUJANGASANA (COBRA POSE)

Lie on abdomen, legs stretched out. Place palms on floor by the side of the chest, forehead resting on ground. Loosen the body.

Slowly raise the head and shoulders and take the head backward as far as possible. Now try to curve the back in circular form till hands are straight.

Ensure that there is no undue stress on the spine. Raise the body above solar plexus. Stay in this position for some time. Slowly return to the original position.

Breathe in while raising the body. Keep breath inside during the last stage of exercise. Breathe out while returning to the original position.

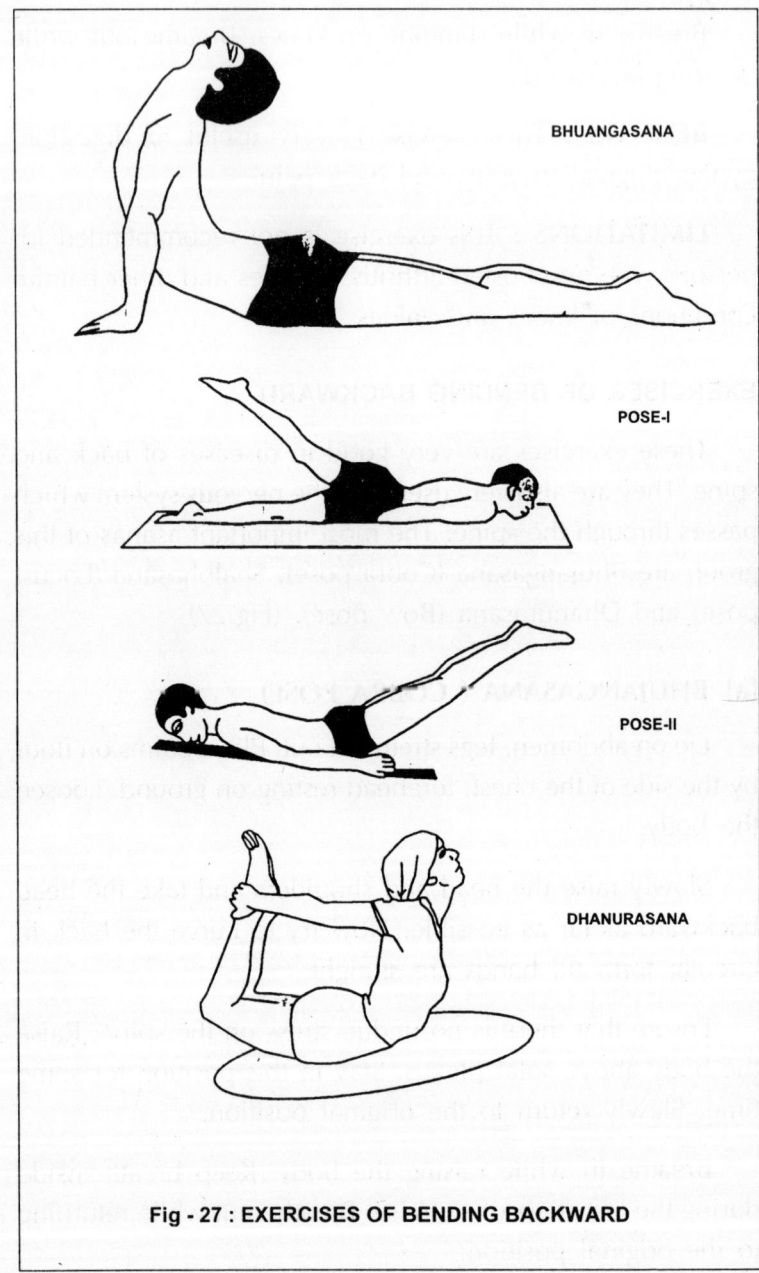

Fig - 27 : EXERCISES OF BENDING BACKWARD

LIMITATIONS : Root canal and central canal stenosis.

BENEFITS : Muscular back pain, Ankylosing spondylitis. Strengthening of cervical and lumbar spine.

[b] SALABHASANA (LOCUST POSTURE)

(i) Lie flat on ground with face downwards. Keep hands on the side of the body with palms under the thighs. Rest the chin on the ground by raising the head.

Keeping one leg straight on the ground, raise the other leg as high as possible. Stay in this position for sometime and bring the leg down slowly. Repeat this action with the other leg.

Breathe in while lying on the ground. Hold the breath while raising the leg and holding it in that position. Breathe out while bringing the leg down. Repeat 5-10 times

(ii) Keep hands under the thighs with the fingers clenched into fists. Rest the chin on the ground by raising the head. Inhale and stiffen the body by pressing the fists against the floor. Slowly raise the legs as high as possible. Keep the legs in straight line while two thighs, knees and ankles touch each other. Weight of the legs must be on body and hands. Retain the posture for sometime and return back to the original position. Breathe in while lying on the floor. Hold the breath while raising the legs and holding it in that position. Breathe out while lowering the legs to the floor.

LIMITATIONS : Peptic ulcer, hernia and acute heart disease, osteo-arthritis of spine. Severe & acute condition of pelvis and sacroiliac joint.

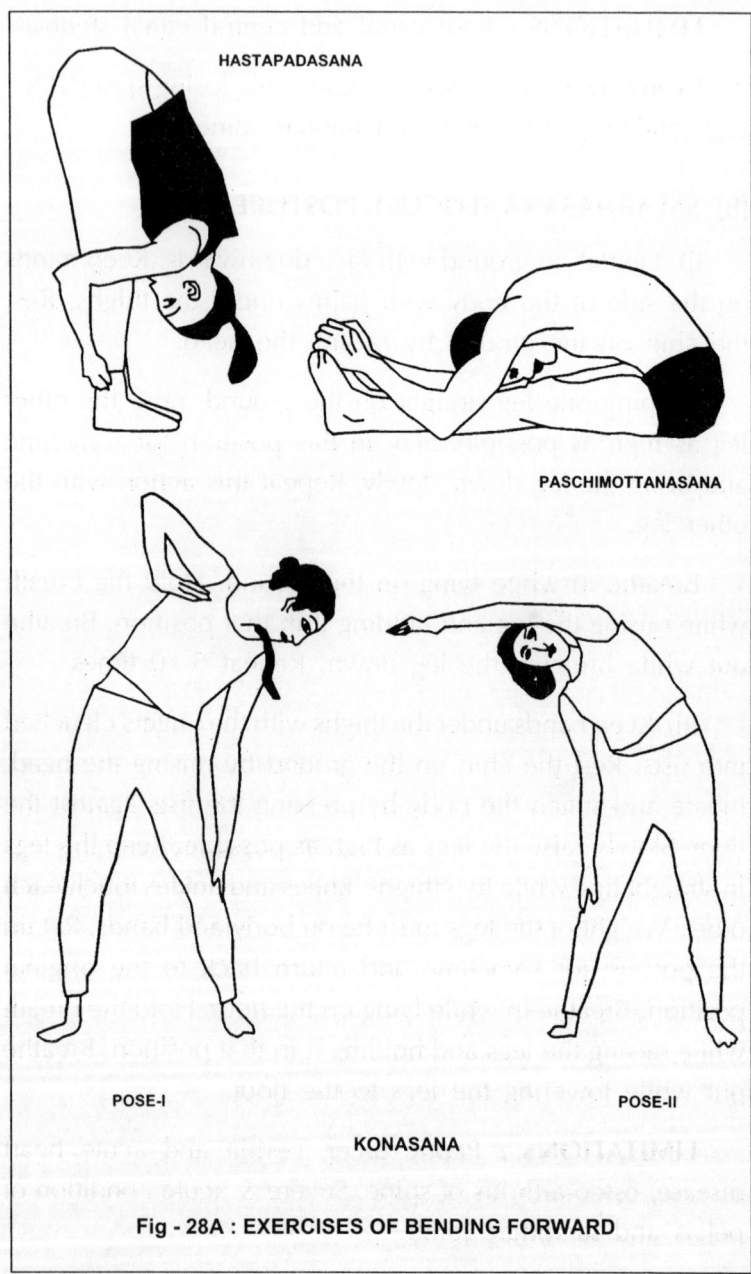

Fig - 28A : EXERCISES OF BENDING FORWARD

Treatment of Arthritis 111

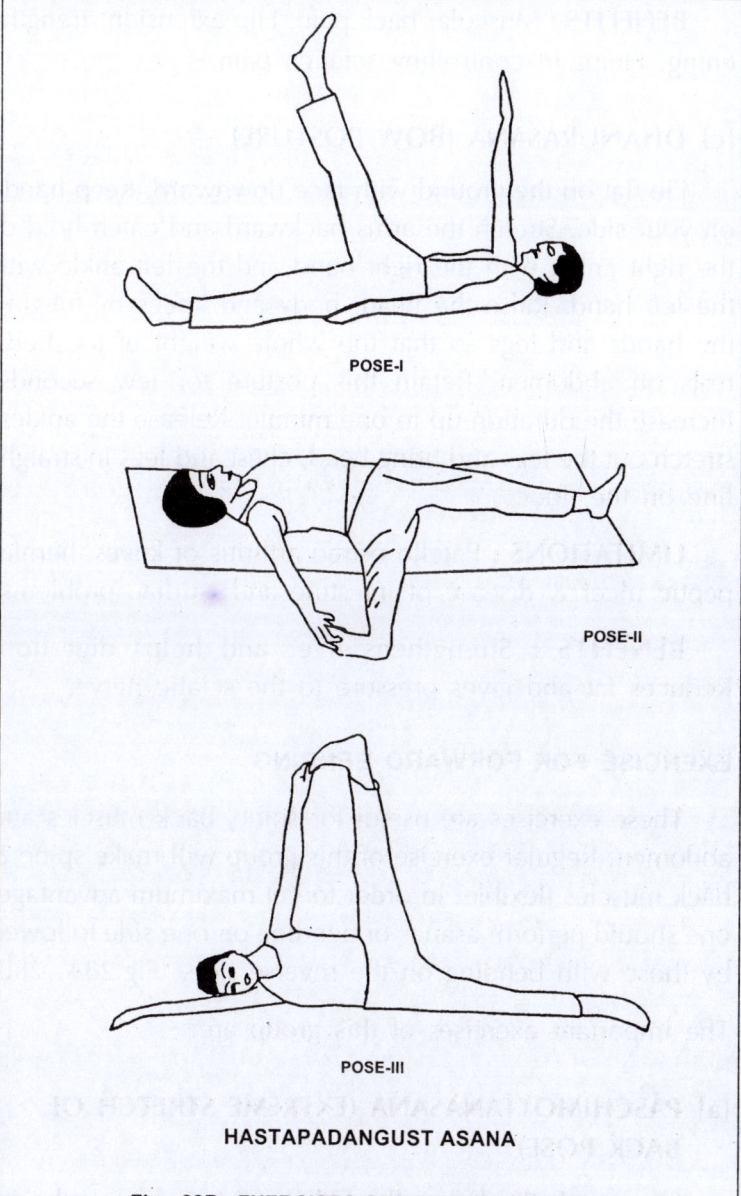

POSE-I

POSE-II

POSE-III

HASTAPADANGUST ASANA

Fig - 28B : EXERCISES OF FORWARD BENDING

BENEFITS : Muscular back pain. Hip extension strengthening. Helps in controlling sciatica pain.

[c] DHANURASANA (BOW POSTURE)

Lie flat on the ground with face downward. Keep hands on your side. Stretch the arms backward and catch hold of the right ankle with the right hand and the left ankle with the left hand. Raise the head, body and knees by tugging the hands and legs so that the whole weight of the body rests on abdomen. Retain this posture for few seconds. Increase the duration up to one minute. Release the ankles, stretch out the legs and bring head, chest and legs in straight line on the floor.

LIMITATIONS : Patello ostreo arthritis of knees, hernia, peptic ulcer & disease of intestine and cardiac problems.

BENEFITS : Strengthens liver and helps digestion. Reduces fat and gives pressure to the sciatic nerve.

EXERCISE FOR FORWARD BENDING

These exercises are useful for spine, back muscles and abdomen. Regular exercise of this group will make spine & back muscles flexible. In order to get maximum advantage, one should perform asanas of bending on one side followed by those with bending on the reverse side. (Fig.28A, 28B)

The important exercises of this group are:

[a] PASCHIMOTTANASANA (EXTREME STRETCH OF BACK POSE)

Sit, stretch the legs fully with toe inwards. Breathe in. Breathing out, bend forward and touch the toes, with hands out stretched. Now touch the knees with the head, drop elbows. Retain this position for about 6 seconds. Inhaling, return to the starting position.

LIMITATIONS : Gross osteo-arthritis of knees, Acute disc prolapse.

BENEFITS : Stiff back and cramp in back muscles. Elasticity of spine is increased. The hamstring muscles behind knees are strengthened. It tones up kidneys and abdominal organs.

[b] HASTAPADASANA (HEAD AND FOOT POSE)

Stand erect, knees straight and feet together. Inhale for 3 seconds. Raise arms above the head till slightly backward. Breathing out for 3 seconds bend forward. Hold ankles with hands and head facing downward. Maintain this position for 6 seconds. Inhaling for 3 seconds return to the starting position.

LIMITATIONS : Resolving & acute disc prolapse and very painful spine and also in cardiac & severe abdominal problems.

BENEFITS : Ankylosing spondylitis and in resolved disc prolapsed.

[c] KONASANA (ANGLE POSE)

Stand erect with feet approximately two feet apart. Keep left hand on waist. Turn head towards right. Keeping the back straight, bend towards the right in such a way that the right hand slides towards the right ankle and the left hand moves up towards the armpit. Repeat on the other side. Breathe normally while standing straight and exhale when bending. Breathe in while coming to normal position.

LIMITATIONS : Resolving and acute disc prolapse. Very painful back. Gross osteo-arthritis of spine and cervical area. Gross osteo-arthritis of knees. Vertigo, hypertension and severe cardiac problems.

BENEFITS : Muscular pains of shoulder girdle, lumbar and cervical. Ankylosing spondyilitis.

- KONASANA – 2 (ANGLE POSE)

Stand erect with the two feet apart. Raise arm above the head touching the ear. Bend side ways to the left and bring right arm parallel to the ground. Slide left arm towards the ankle and remain in this position for sometime. Repeat on other side.

While standing breathe normally. Bending sideways breathe out. Inhale while coming to normal position. Limitations & benefits as in Konasana – 1.

[d] HASTAPADANGUSHTASANA (HAND, LEG & TOE POSE)

Pose - 1 Lie on back with feet straight. Inhaling for 3 seconds hold right arm up. Exhaling for 3 seconds raise right leg towards right hand. Hold this position for 5 seconds. Inhaling for 3 seconds return to the normal position. Repeat it on the other side.

LIMITATIONS : Gross osteo-arthritis of hip and acute disc prolapse. Hypertension, cardiac problems, pregnancy and hernia.

BENEFITS : Muscular pains, osteo-arthritis of knees and ankylosing spondylitis.

Pose - 2 Lie on the back with the feet straight, keep arms in 'T' position. Exhaling take right leg side ways as far as possible till it touches the hand. Stay in this position for 6 seconds and come back to normal position inhaling. Repeat in opposite side.

LIMITATIONS : Gross osteo-arthritis of hip. Acute lumber disc prolapse.

BENEFITS : Muscular pains and all spine problems.

Pose - 3 Lie on right side. Inhale and raise the left hand. Now exhale and raise the left leg side way at 90^0 stay in this position for 6 seconds. Inhale and return to original position. Turn other side and repeat.

LIMITATIONS : Gross osteo-arthritis of the hip and acute lumbar disc prolapse.

BENEFITS : Osteo-arthritis of knees, problems of spine.

SURYA NAMASKAR

Surya namaskar is a combined process of Yogasana and Pranayama (Yogic exercises and regulated breathing). (Fig.29A, 29B) This exercise reduces abdominal fat, makes limbs and spine flexible and increases breathing capacity. There are twelve spinal positions each stretching different ligaments and giving different movement to vertebral column. It gives mild exercise to leg and arm muscles and ensures good circulation of blood. It is a boon to persons with stiff spine and limbs.

During different positions, movement of limbs and breathing must be very slow and rhythmical. Inhalation and ex-

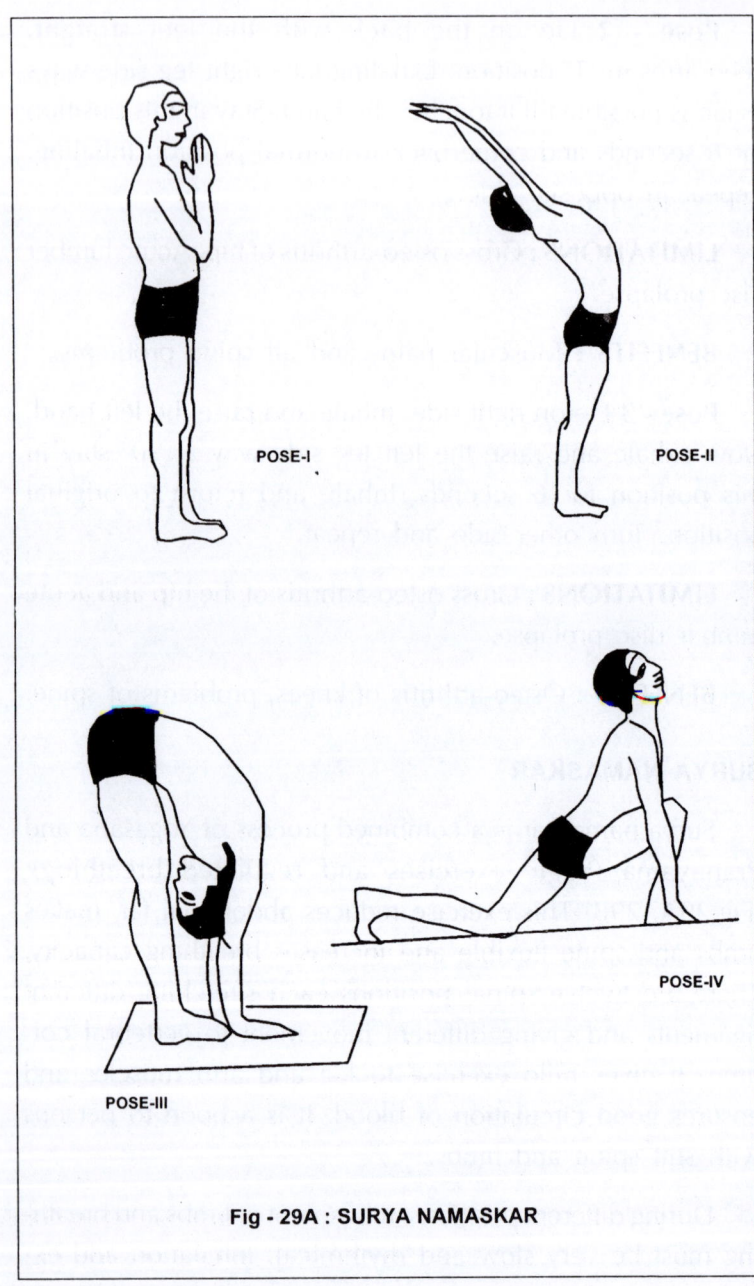

Fig - 29A : SURYA NAMASKAR

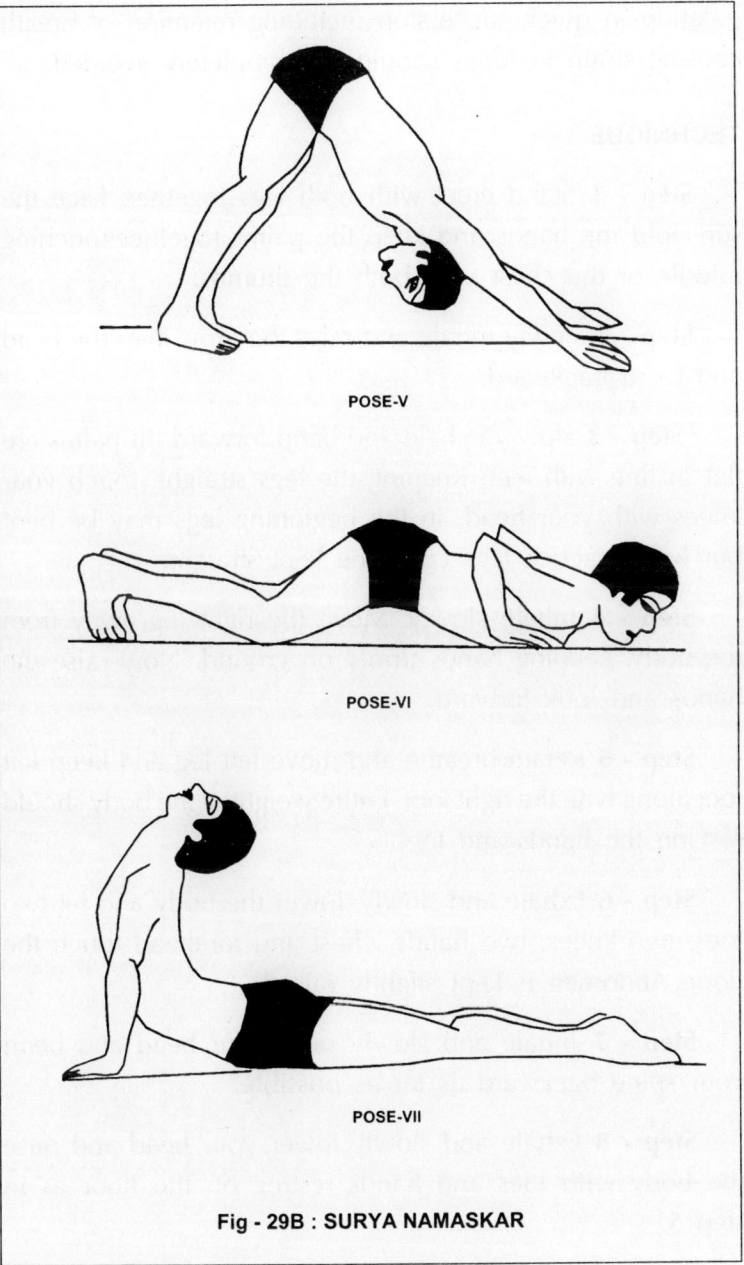

POSE-V

POSE-VI

POSE-VII

Fig - 29B : SURYA NAMASKAR

halation in quick succession including retention of breath causing strain in lungs should be completely avoided.

TECHNIQUE :

Step - 1 Stand erect with both legs together. Face the sun, fold the hands and keep the palms together touching middle of the chest with both the thumbs.

Step - 2 Slowly inhale and raise the arms over the head and bend backward.

Step - 3 Slowly exhale and bend forward till palms are flat in line with feet. Keeping the legs straight, touch your knees with your head. In the beginning legs may be bent but with practice legs could be kept straight.

Step - 4 Inhale slowly. Move the right leg away from the body, keeping hands firmly on ground. Now raise the hands and look forward.

Step - 5 Retain breathe and move left leg and keep left foot along with the right foot. Entire weight of the body should rest on the hands and toes.

Step - 6 Exhale and slowly, lower the body and let two toes, two knees, two hands, chest and forehead touch the floor. Abdomen is kept slightly raised.

Step - 7 Inhale and slowly raise your head and bend your spine backward as far as possible.

Step - 8 Exhale and slowly lower your head and raise the body with toes and hands resting on the floor as in step 5.

Step - 9 Inhale and bring left foot along the level of the hands. Right foot and knee should touch the ground. Look forward as in step 4.

Step - 10 Exhale and bring right leg also forward and come as in step 3.

Step - 11 Inhale and raise hands overhead and bend back ward as in step 2.

Step - 12 Slowly bring your hands as in step 1. Exhale and relax.

EXERCISES FOR PRAYER (See Fig.30)

[a] PADMASANA (LOTUS POSE)

Sit on floor with legs fully stretched out, keep spine and neck erect. Bend right leg at knee and place the foot on the left thigh with palm facing up. Now bend the left leg at knee and place the foot on right thigh with palm facing up. Place two hands with palm facing up on respective knee joints. Bend index finger and it should touch the middle portion of the thumb. Keep eyes closed and breathe normally.

LIMITATIONS : This exercise is not suitable for persons having gross osteo-arthritis of knees.

BENEFITS : It is a stretching exercise. It improves blood circulation in lower portion of spine and stomach.

[b] SUKHASANA

Sit with legs stretched. Bend right leg and put it below the left thigh. Now bend the left leg and put it below the

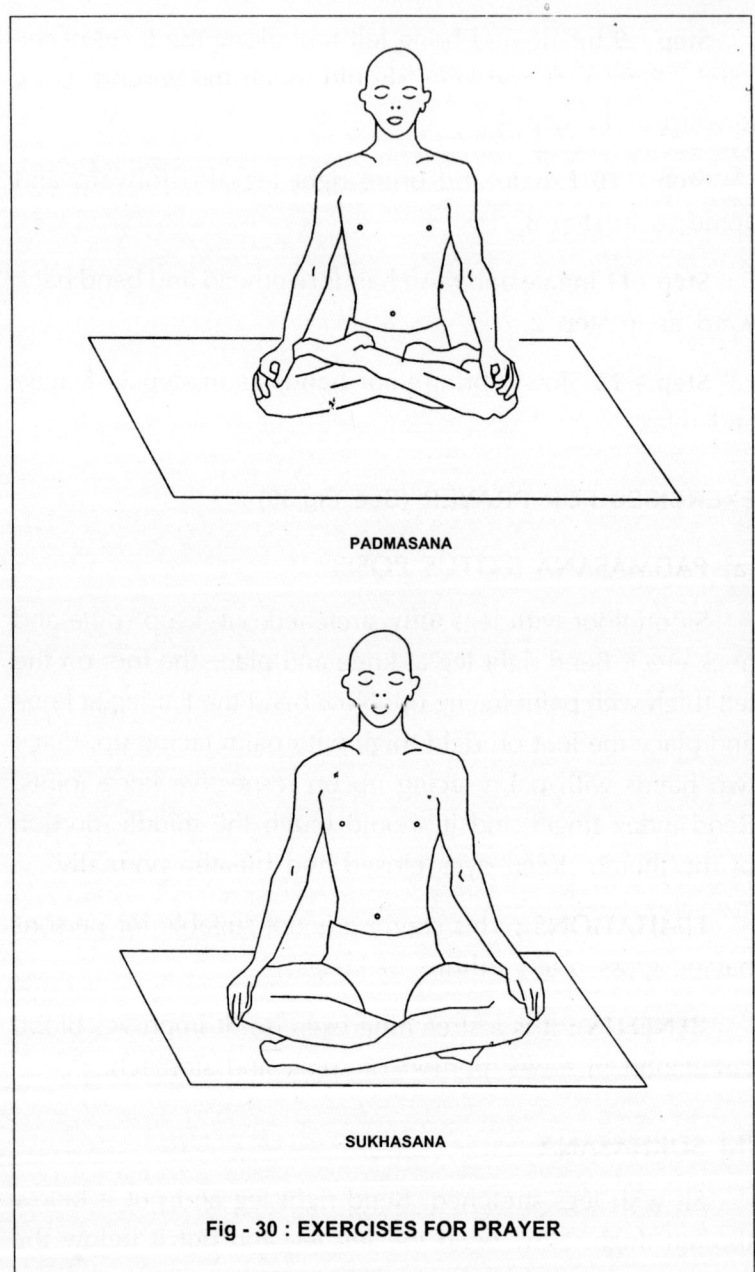

Fig - 30 : EXERCISES FOR PRAYER

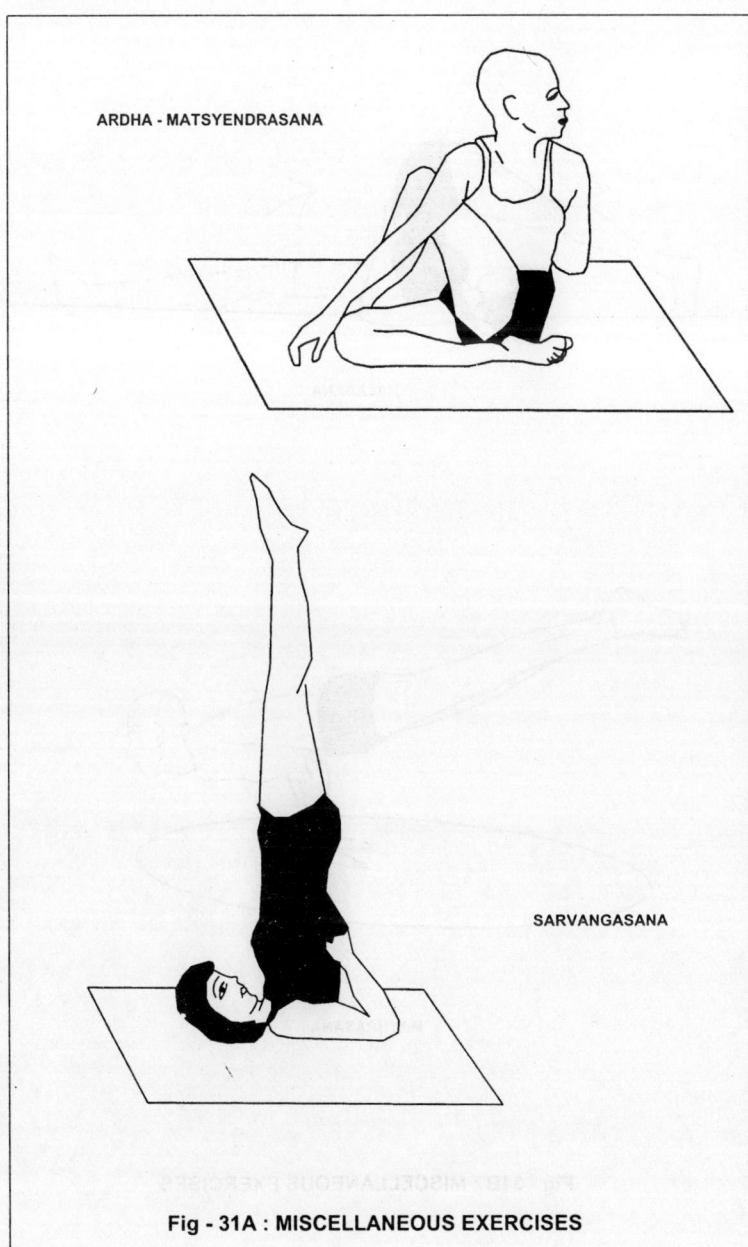

Fig - 31A : MISCELLANEOUS EXERCISES

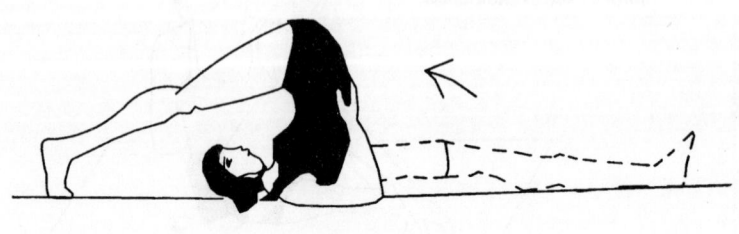

HALASANA

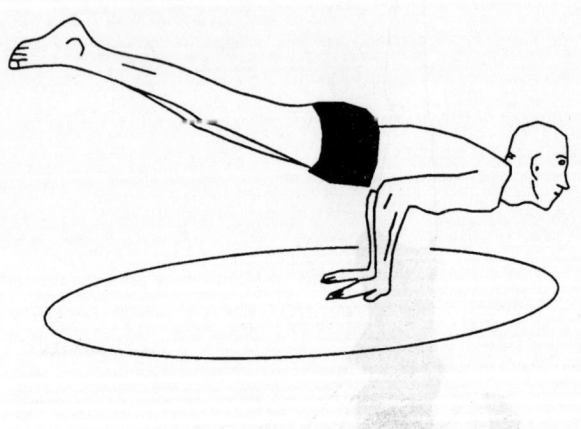

MAYURASANA

Fig - 31B : MISCELLANEOUS EXERCISES

right thigh. Keep hands on your knees and keep the head, neck and back straight.

This is a simple exercise and is ideal for less experienced people.

MISCELLENEOUS EXERCISES

[a] ARDHA – MATSYENDRASANA

Sit down with feet spread in front. Bend left leg placing left foot besides right hip. Place right foot on outside of left knee, keeping foot flat on ground. Bring left arm and place it outside the right knee, elbow at knee and left hand grasping right foot circle the right hand behind the back and twist the trunk towards right as much as possible. Hold this position for 6 seconds. Return to starting position and repeat in other direction. (Fig.31A)

Exhale while bending the back. Hold the breathe in the last stage. Inhale while returning to the starting position.

BENEFITS : General muscular pain and stiffness. It improves the functioning of pancreas and kidney.

[b] SARVANGASANA (ALL LIMB POSTURE)

Spread thick blanket on floor and lie flat over it with legs stretched out, heels and knees together and hands close to the side of the body, palm facing the floor. Slowly inhale and raise the legs without bending the knees. Slowly lift the trunk and support it with your hands bent at the elbow. Keep the spine vertical. The back of shoulders, neck and the back of the crown of head should touch the floor and chin should be pressed against the chest. Keep this position with normal breathing.

Exhale slowly lower the legs without jerk and release the position of head. Slowly slide down and lie flat.

LIMITATIONS : Cervical spondilytis.chronic eye disease.High and low blood pressure.

BENEFITS : During the practice of this asana every part of body is given exercise. Circulation of blood is directed to thyroid and para thyroid glands. It strengthens muscles of cervical region. It also helps the persons with varicose veins.

[c] HALASANA (PLOUGH POSTURE)

Lie flat on your back with arms on the side and palm resting on ground. Keep your legs together. Raise legs slowly without bending knees till they are at right angle with trunk. Keeping hand on ground raise hip and lumbar portion of the back and bring down legs to the floor beyond the head. Press the chin against the chest and breathe slowly. Remain in this posture for 6 seconds. Slowly raise legs and bring them gradually to the original position. (Fig. 31B)

LIMITATIONS : Cervical spondylitis.

BENEFITS : The asana reduces excess fat from abdomen, thighs and hips. It cures various complications of back, spine and shoulders.

[d] MAYURASANA (PEACOCK POSTURE)

Kneel on the floor with knees slightly apart and toes resting on ground. Bend the body forward, join arms together and rest the palms on the floor with two little fingers touching each other and all fingers pointing towards the feet. (Fig.31B)

Slowly bend forward and rest the abdomen on the elbows and chest on the upper part of the arms. Stretch the legs backward and keep them stiff. Balance your body parallel to the ground and remain in this position at least for 6 seconds. Release from the pose, first lower the head and then legs. Place the knees by the side of the hands and then release the position of the hands. Lie flat on theground and relax.

BENEFITS : This asana strengthens forearms, elbows, wrists and removes a number of abdomen diseases. It increases digestive power, tones up stomach, kidney & spleen. It is beneficial for those suffering from diabetes.

and rest the hands on the floor with the little fingers touching each other. Inhale through the nose and exhale. Repeat at least six times.

SUGGESTION: If you find it difficult to assume the above position, stretch the lower part of the arms, stretch the legs back also and lift them stiff. Balance your body, keeping only the ground and chin in the position, at least for a second. Relax and bring the toes first down, the head and then legs. Lift the knees to the side of the hands and then release the position of the hands are flat on the ground and relax.

BENEFITS: This asana, when others' postures above, while also removes a number of abdominal diseases. It also increases appetite. It tones up stomach, kidney & spleen. It is beneficial for those suffering from diabetes.

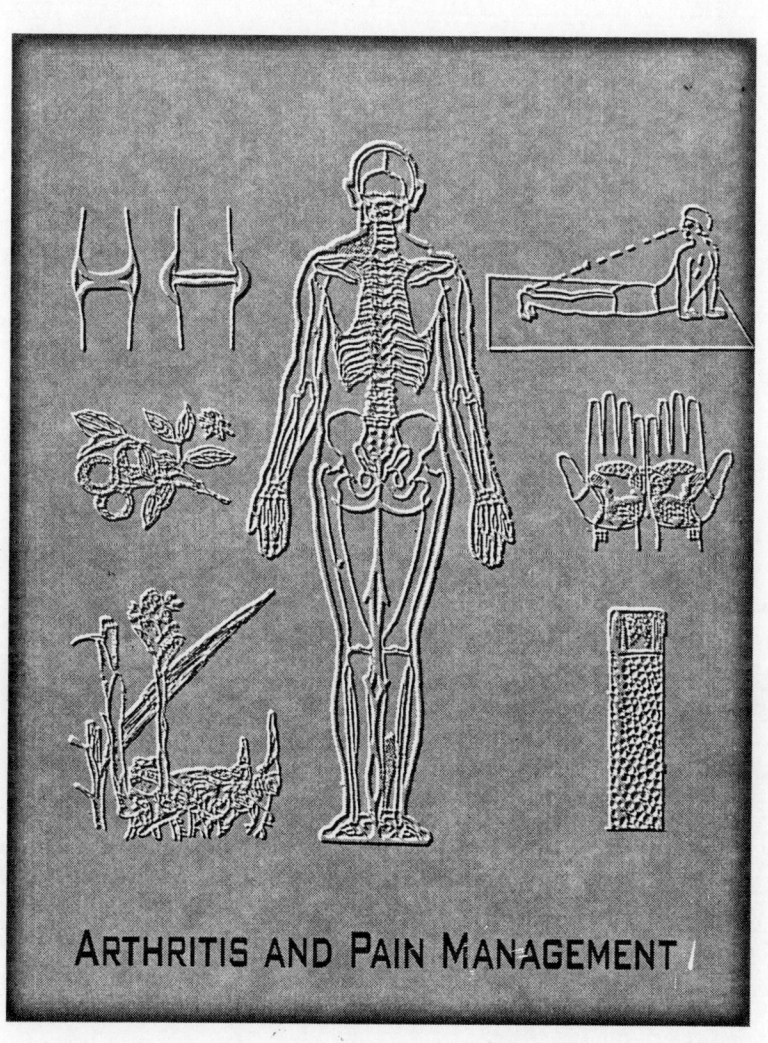

ARTHRITIS AND PAIN MANAGEMENT

Chapter

3

ARTHRITIS AND PAIN MANAGEMENT

3.1 INTRODUCTION

In arthritis there is pain, inflammation and stiffness in joints. The pain in the joint varies enormously in quality and severity from sharp stabbing sensation, burning sensation to grinning pain. However, pain is always there.

Chronic pain is persistent and not intermittent. It is severe at times while it is dull at other times. However, it reminds you of its presence all the time. It may last for months and years and not for days and weeks. Different forms of arthritis produce chronic pain.

We usually create situations ourselves, which aggravate chronic pain further. Some of these are

 i. Luxurious but stressful life causes muscle tension.
 ii. Fear and anxiety causes contraction and muscle spasm.
 iii. Negative frame of mind, stresses at work place, strains in inter personal relations and financial problems etc also cause muscle spasm.

iv. Muscles are main shock absorbers of our body. They deload joints and keep them mobile. Muscle harmony is crucial for proper functioning of joints. Lack of exercise causes muscle dysfunction and increases their wear and tear.

Usually the treatment of pain is based on the assumption that the underlying physical cause must be found out and corrected. This theory is useful when we have to treat an acute pain but when the pain becomes chronic, the treatment should not be confined to pain only but to person as a whole i.e. his suffering, his behavior and the environment around him. After treating all these factors, one will find that the pain is not such an obstacle as one thinks and can be managed successfully.

3.2 DIFFERENT STEPS FOR PAIN MANAGEMENT

❖ **Step – 1**

CONTROLLING SEVERE PAIN & INFLAMMATION

When the pain or pain with inflammation is severe and unbearable, it is necessary to resort to medication. Immediate relief is usually obtained with painkiller and anti-inflammatory drugs. As has been mentioned in chapter 2.2, the allopathic pain killers and anti-inflammatory drugs usually have side effects. However, in severe pain when one needs immediate relief one should take the pain killer or anti-inflammatory drug, which is relatively safe.

Depending on symptoms, homeopathic medicines should be used for reducing pain and inflammation. In addition to pathology, different symptoms accompanying pain are used for the selection of medicine. These medicines are very useful and in long run they have positive effect on the body constitution. They also help in curing the disease. The details of different homeopathic medicines used in the treatment of arthritis is given in chapter 2, section 4.

Ayurvedic medicines used for controlling pain and inflammation are discussed in chapter 2, section 5.

For best management of pain and inflammatory conditions one should judiciously use the above methods. If pain is very severe one can use painkiller for a short-time. Simultaneously one should use homeopathic and ayurvedic medicines and acupressure techniques to reduce pain further. It is possible to reduce pain substantially and manage it with the use of homeopathic & ayurvedic medicines and acupressure techniques only which have no side effects.

In extremely severe conditions when it is not possible to manage pain with the help of different systems of medicine, one can take recourse to injections into joints or to surgery as discussed in chapter 2 section 2. However, it should be mentioned here that use of injections or surgical method as a treatment of arthritis should be used as a last resort only.

Besides, the medication, the application of heat is very comforting. For this purpose one can use hot water bottles and infrared devices etc. Heat promotes better circulation around injured or sore part of the body. A warm bath or shower can bring relief and help in promoting relaxation. In some cases cold spray or ice packs can bring lot of relief.

By experimenting one can find whether cold or warm application suits you. At times gentle pressure, hard pressure or massage ameliorates and should be used.

❖ Step – 2

SETTING NERVOUS SYSTEM IN ORDER

Set the central nervous system passing through the spinal cord in order. The procedure to set central nervous system in order is given in section 5 of chapter 2.

❖ Step – 3

CONDITIONS THAT AGGRAVATE PAIN

Certain conditions, which aggravate pain in arthritis, should be tackled next. These include:

- Constipation
- Certain foods
- Obesity

Different ways to tackle these conditions are given in previous chapters. We shall review them here

[a] CONSTIPATION

In order to control constipation the following steps should be taken,

i. Set solar plexus in order. Different methods in this regard are given in chapter 2, section 3.

ii. Person should develop a habit of taking food at regular intervals. Raw, fresh foods with lots of fibers are good for health. The details about the food is given in chapter 2, section 3.

iii. Take two glasses of lukewarm water in the morning and do the following yogic exercises 8 – 10 times

Tadasana (Palm tree pose)
- Triyak Tadasana (Curved palm tree pose)
- Kati-Chakrasana (Circular movement of back)
- Triyak Bhujangasana (Curved snake pose)
- Crow movement

The details regarding these exercises is given in chapter 2, section 6.

In Chronic cases of constipation purgatives can be taken for a short time. Caster oil is one of the best purgatives. Very good results have been obtained by use of the following.

- TREPHALA - This powder is available in all ayurvedic stores. Take one tablespoon of this powder in one glass water. Keep it overnight. Next morning filter it with thin clean piece of cloth and drink it.
- ISAPGOL - It has high soluble fiber content and is used to prevent constipation. Take one spoon of this powder and drink with lukewarm water in the night before sleeping.

One can take trephala and isapgol on alternate days.

- There are certain medicines in homeopathy, which control the condition of constipation. Based on matching of symptoms, medicines can be selected. The details of these medicine are given in chapter 2, section 4.

- Pressure on certain points help in controlling constipation. The details of these points is given in chapter 2, section 5.

[b] CERTAIN FOOD

Certain foods are heavy to digest, produce gastric conditions in stomach and aggravate pain. Persons with arthritis should avoid following foods.

i. Sour curd
ii. Vegetables like Lady's finger, Pumpkin, Jack fruit, Cauliflower etc. Tomato is also harmful.
iii. Oily and sour foods.
iv. Large quantity of tea, coffee and liquor.
v. Chewing and smoking tobacco.
vi. Green and red chilies.
vii. The intake of all pulses except moong should be restricted.
viii. Intake of peas and gram should also be restricted.

There are certain spices, which are very useful. They include black pepper, ginger, cardamom, cinnamon, cloves, cumin seeds and turmeric etc.

[c] OBESITY

In persons with arthritis, being obese puts more stress on the joints and hence it aggravates the painful condition.

The ideal weight of a person is given in table 1.

TABLE - 1

Ideal weight of Men and Women after 25 year of age - **'Men'**

Height in cm	Small frame Weight in Kg.	Medium frame Weight in Kg.	Large frame Weight in Kg.
152	45.4 – 48.4	49.4 – 53.0	52.0 – 56.2
155	47.0 – 51.0	50.0 – 54.3	53.5 – 58.0
157	48.6 – 52.0	51.9 – 55.6	54.3 – 58.8
160	49.8 – 53.9	53.0 – 57.0	56.9 – 60.9
163	51.4 – 55.6	54.3 – 58.8	59.2 – 64.1
165	52.7 – 56.8	55.9 – 60.0	59.2 – 64.1
168	54.3 – 57.4	57.6 – 61.6	60.9 – 66.1
170	55.6 – 60.0	59.2 – 63.7	62.5 – 67.8
173	57.2 – 61.6	60.9 – 65.3	64.1 – 69.4
175	58.8 – 63.3	62.5 – 67.0	65.7 – 71.4
178	60.4 – 65.0	64.1 – 68.6	67.4 – 73.5
180	62.0 – 67.0	65.7 – 70.6	69.0 – 75.5
183	63.6 – 68.6	67.4 – 72.2	70.4 – 77.2

'Women'

147	42.5 – 45.3	44.9 – 48.2	47.8 – 51.9
150	42.9 – 46.1	45.7 – 49.0	48.6 – 52.7
152	43.7 – 47.0	46.5 – 49.8	48.6 – 52.7
155	44.9 – 48.2	47.7 – 51.0	50.6 – 55.1
157	46.1 – 49.4	49.0 – 52.3	51.9 – 56.3
160	47.4 – 51.0	50.6 – 53.9	53.5 – 58.0
163	48.6 – 52.3	51.9 – 55.1	54.3 – 59.2
165	50.2 – 53.9	53.1 – 57.2	56.3 – 61.2
168	51.4 – 55.5	54.3 – 58.8	58.0 – 62.9

If a person has weight more than 10% of the ideal weight, he is said to be obese and he should try to bring his weight near the ideal weight.

People usually put on weight by eating more food than needed. However, not all over weight persons eat more than a normal person. In these types of persons obesity is genetic rather than an abnormality. Not much is known about factors responsible for this type of obesity. When these type of persons reduce calorie intake for reducing weight, instead of their weight going down their body temperature goes down.

The other types of obesity are due to

i. The tumors, injury, inflammation with meningitis at times cause hypothalamic obesity.

ii. Hypothyroid causes weight gain in spite of strict dieting.

iii. Over secretion of adrenal gland.

iv. Changes in sex gland function such as castration and menopause.

v. Certain drugs such as estrogens used in contraceptive pills and phenothiazine used in psychiatry are also associated with weight gain.

However, these causes of obesity are not very common and consultation with doctor is required to control them.

In order to control weight one should use low calorie balanced diet. Exercise along with proper diet is the best way to loose weight but not the muscle tissues. However, exercise should be chosen as per your age and in consultation with your doctor. In case of arthritis walking is the best form of exercise.

Most of the obese persons will benefit from the above however for some persons it would be necessary to take an expert help.

More than slimming it is important to stay slim and healthy. Diet selection, exercise and continuity are essential for any long term slimming programme. One should select diet as per his choice in consultation with his doctor.

- *OBESITY AND HOMEOPATHY*

If obesity is due to some disease, it is necessary that it should be diagnosed and based on its symptoms, medicine is given. However, in other cases the best medicine to control obesity is the constitutional medicine.

- *OBESITY AND ACUPRESSURE*

In order to control weight, pressure should be applied to the points corresponding to thyroid and parathyroid, adrenal, stomach, intestine and kidneys. In addition, points corresponding to sex organs should also be pressed.

❖ **Step – 4**

CORRECTING POSTURE

The bad posture can cause pain or aggravate the same. The examples of bad postures are:
  i. Driving long distance on a badly designed seat.
  ii. House wives using kitchen of wrong height.

iii. Hairdressers and dentists standing for a long period exerting a strain on neck, shoulders and arm muscles.
iv. In super market checkout staff has to make movement on one side of counter only.
v. Even at home, sitting for hours watching T.V. or reading books without proper head or back support.
vi. In office doing routine file work with neck in one position.

Any one who maintains one position for a longtime or has bad pasture is likely to have muscular spasm from excessive tension. Bad posture is also the main reason of neck pain. Sitting or standing in slouched position flattens the normal cervical curvature in the neck; putting a strain on all the muscles supporting the head. Sleeping with high pillow has the same affect.

Bad posture may be due to injury. In persons with chronic pain, the posture suffers in the process of finding the least painful position. This will result in various muscle groups in the body under tension and aggravating pain in the muscle group under strain.

- **CORRECTING THE POSTURE**

In cases of bad posture, correcting the posture will improve frequency and severity of pain. The exercises designed to tone and strengthen the muscles will also be more effective after improvement of posture.

The choice of well-designed chair is especially important if you sit for a longtime at your work. The chair should be strong and solid enough to take your weight and should not

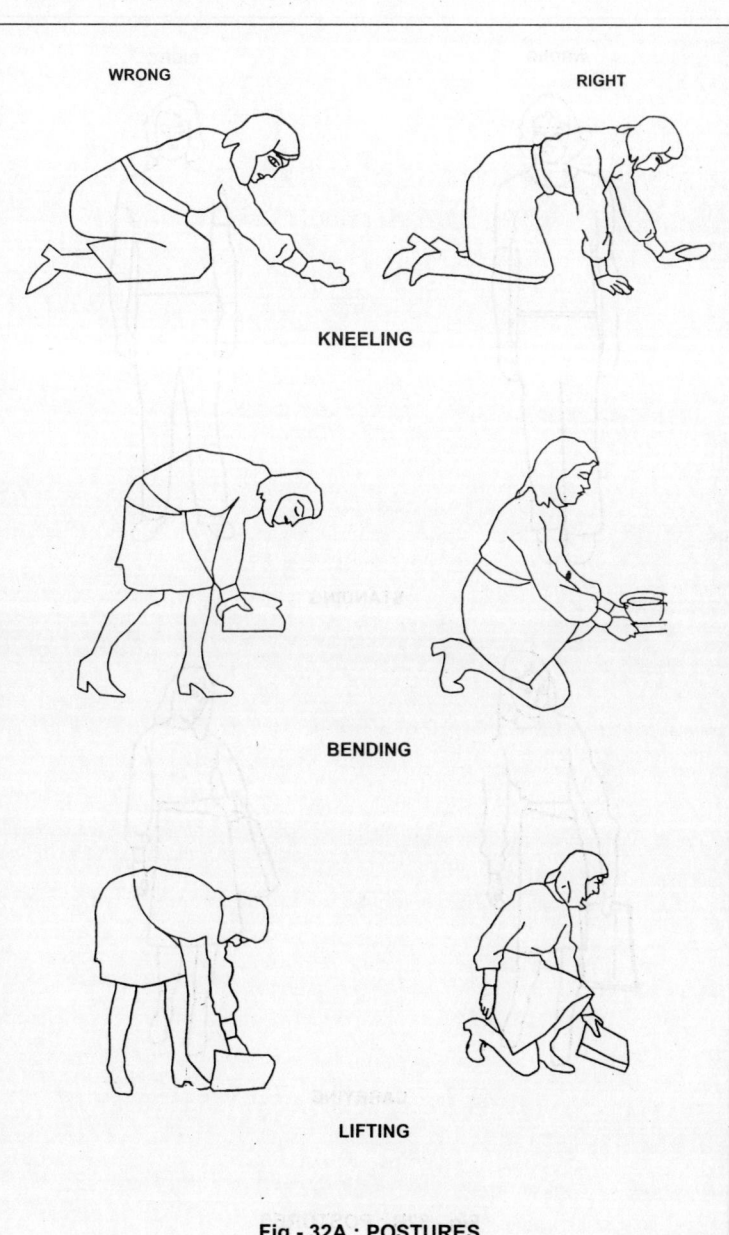

Fig - 32A : POSTURES

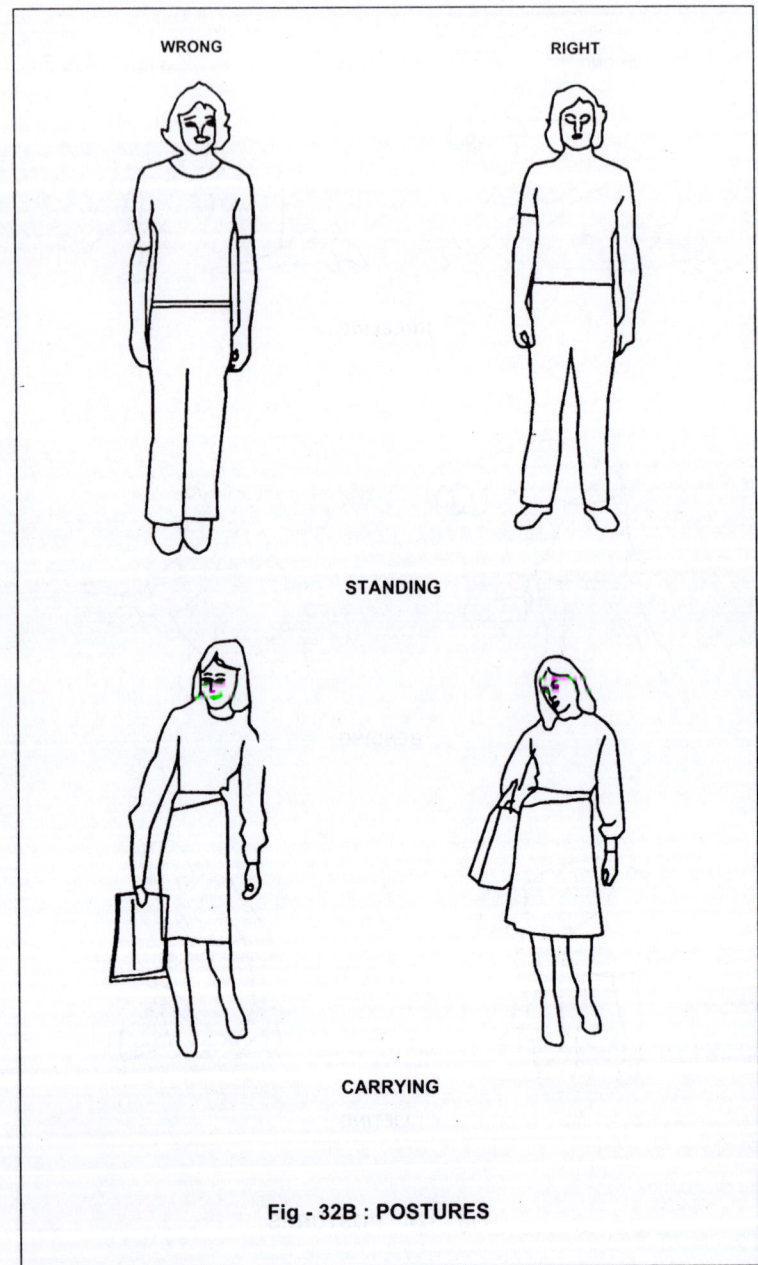

Fig - 32B : POSTURES

sag when you sit in it. The chair should be comfortable and should give sufficient support to your back. Sit squarely with both feet on the floor a short distance in front of your chair. Do not sit one leg over the other or wrapping one leg round the leg of the chair.

- AVOIDING BACK TROUBLE

Discs of cartilage separate the bones of the spinal column, which allow the bones to bend in any direction. The more the spine bends, greater is the strain on discs. If the spine is bent and at the same time compressed as when one lifts heavy weight, the discs maybe squeezed and deformed. The protrusion of disc causes trouble when it presses spinal cord or the nerve running through it. To prevent back trouble it is important to keep spine as upright as possible in all lifting movements. When the nerve is pressed, it causes pain in the area of the body served by it.

- CORRECTING HEAD AND NECK POSITION

Correcting head and neck position is very simple. While sitting, standing and walking, your chin should remain parallel to floor. In case there is tension in shoulders, allow them to relax and drop. There is generally a tendency to lower the head while reading or writing, it puts strain on the back of neck.

- CORRECT WAY OF GETTING OUT OF SEAT

Learning to get out of seat will reduce strain on your body. Use your arms and move your body towards the edge of the seat. Still sitting, place one foot slightly forward and

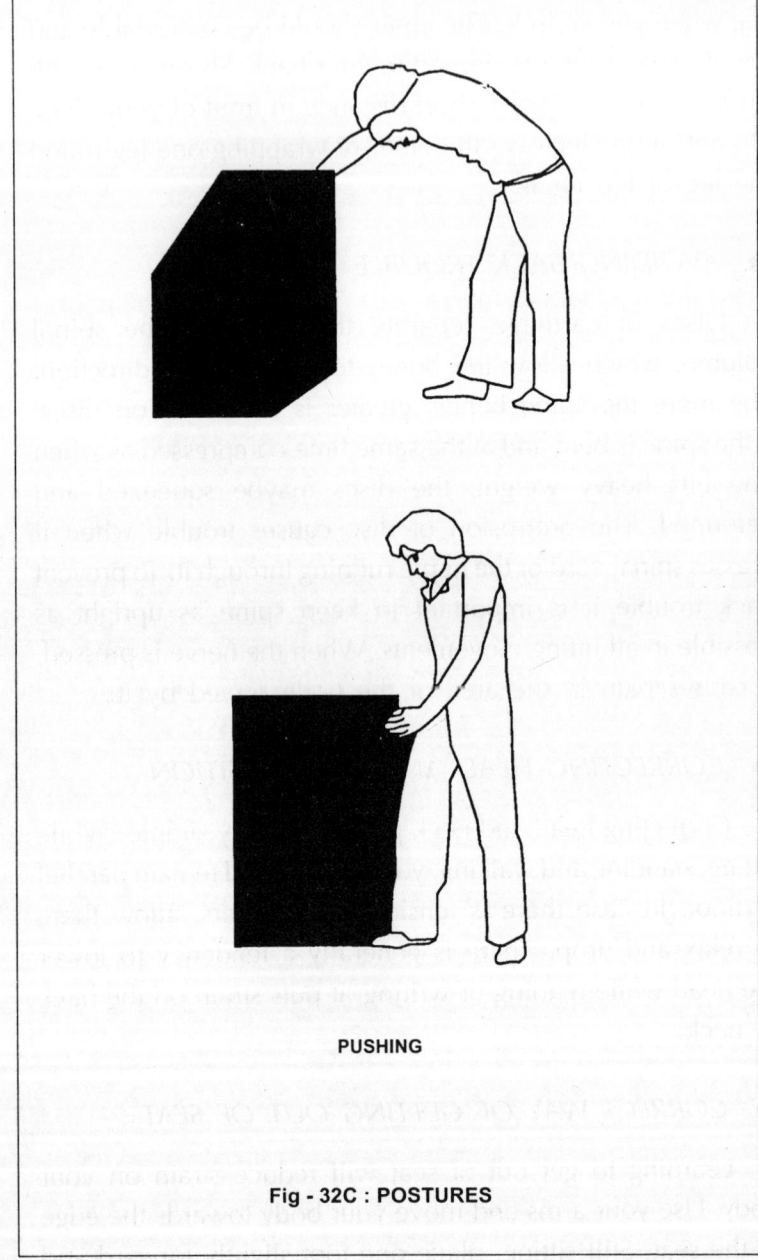

PUSHING

Fig - 32C : POSTURES

taking weight on both the feet and then rise. Initially you can use your hands by putting them on knees while sitting.

- CORRECT WAY OF SLEEPING

In case you have chronic pain, one should sleep in a posture, which is suitable to your condition. Persons with neck and head pain should not use high pillow. Japanese type pillow (Shaped like a dog bone) is very suitable for this condition. People with leg and back pain can be helped by sleeping on one side with upper leg drawn up to knee level and resting on a pillow.

❖ Step – 5

EXERCISE

This is one of the most important steps in managing pain and rehabilitation of a person. In case of severe inflammation and pain in joint, complete rest for a week or two along with acupressure, homeopathic medicine and at times pain killers is recommended. The period of rest should not be open ended and should not be left to the sweet will of the patient. There is generally a tendency on the part of the patient to continue taking rest for a long time. Without exercise muscles become inactive and weak and are likely to go into spasm. This process of weakness takes place very quickly. In persons with chronic pain, this deterioration is faced in the entire body due to reduced level of activity. The condition will further deteriorate with inactivity and efficiency of heart and lungs will be reduced in long run. It is therefore necessary that the condition of the patient should be periodically reviewed by the doctor and a programme of exercises should be prescribed. The exercise will slowly increase mobility, flexibility and circulation. In arthritic sufferers exercise is necessary to strengthen, condition and maintain a range of movement in joints.

Even when one recognises the importance of exercise, one may be tempted to do too much or do the wrong kind of exercises. It can be very harmful as it will increase the level of pain and further convince the person that the pain is linked to the movement. It may result in frustration, anger, irritation and also depression. It will further develop a fear from movement or motophobia. In these type of cases, it will require a great convincing that no harm will come from exercise of the right kind.

Movement is very important for getting fit and managing pain. The exercise stimulates production of endorphins, which are natural painkillers. There are certain principles, which should be followed in an exercise programme e.g.

- In order to select an exercise, take the help of your physiotherapist. In addition to this, certain type of yogic exercises are very useful. The details regarding yogic exercises is given in chapter 2.6.
- Exercise should not involve strain. Right type of yogic exercises is best for this purpose. Over straining should be avoided. However, even gentle exercise may produce some aches and pains, these are not to be taken as a reason for worry.
- One should be regular in exercises and should build strength, stamina and mobility by progressively increasing the exercises.
- Set targets and try to achieve them. Aim at steady progress without over strain. If the target is high, adjust at a comfortable level and build up again.

Depending on the type of problem, a set of yogic exercises is given in chapter 2.6. Persons suffering with arthritis will find different exercises very useful. However, before starting a set of yogic exercises it is necessary to know the right type of exercise and a proper way of doing the same and for this purpose training and advice of an expert is a must.

❖ **Step – 6**

RELAXATION AND STRESS MANAGEMENT

Persons with chronic pain are faced with a typical problem, as the professionals are not in a position to help them fully. They fear that when professionals are not able to help them, they should be beyond help and their pain will never go away. This gives them a feeling of depression, anger and isolation. There is therefore vicious cycle of pain, stress, fear, anxiety, more pain more stress and so on. Tension resulting from this may produce circulation problems arising from decreased blood flow, increased sweat level, digestive problems, pain in shoulders, neck and head etc. Tension results in sleep problems. Tense body increases pain with negative thoughts, which further aggravate pain and are an obstacle to sound sleep.

However in order to overcome these symptoms one should learn to relax effectively.

Relaxation does not mean sleeping, watching T.V. or reading light books. It is a process during which tension is moved away from all muscles and organs of the body and blood flows freely throughout the entire system. Relaxation produces feeling of calmness and brings high blood pressure down, endorphins are produced in large quantities and in the process pain is reduced.

The different methods of relaxation include
a) Physical methods
b) Savasana
c) Pranayam
d) Meditation

[a] PHYSICAL METHOD

During relaxation exercises wear comfortable loose clothing, Cover yourself with a light cloth as during deep relaxation, body temperature goes down.

Basic to all relaxation exercises is the skill of right ways of breathing. There are mainly two types of breathing.
- Breathing through diaphragm
- Breathing through chest

For relaxation purpose deep breathing through diaphragm is most appropriate and is discussed below.

• BREATHING THROUGH DIAPHRAGM

This can be done in the sitting position or lying on the back. Put one hand on your solar plexus. Breathe in deeply. The stomach will inflate and the hand will go up. As the stomach inflates, the area around the heart is pressed down and the lungs will expand.

Now breathe out deeply. In this position the area around stomach is compressed and the hand will go down towards spine. In this position maximum air is subjected out of lungs.

In this exercise do not make any movement in chest and shoulders.

- **EXERCISES FOR MUSCLE RELAXATION**

    EXERCISE – I

    Sit in fully supported position in a chair or lie down on your back. Breathe through diaphragm. When the breath is steady, focus your attention on your arms. Lift the arms and extend them. Breathe in slowly for 5 seconds and simultaneously clench the fist and hold tension in it. Then breathing out let the tension go and allow arms to fall back in resting position. Feel the muscles go slump. Repeat 3 times.

    EXERCISE - II

    Take a deep breath into chest, hold it for 5 seconds tensing the muscles in chest area. Allow the breath and tension to go and relax completely. Repeat 3 times.

    EXERCISE – III

    Lie down on your back and slightly bend knees. Tighten the muscles around abdomen and pelvis area. Breathe in, hold the breath and tension for 5 seconds. Breathe out and release tension. Repeat 3 times.

    EXERCISE – IV

    Sit in fully supported position. Raise the shoulders towards the ears and pull down head towards the ears. Hold breath and tension for 5 seconds. Breathe out and release tension. Repeat 3 times.

EXERCISE - V

Tighten the muscles of the thighs. Take a deep breath, hold the tension for 5 seconds. Breathe out, release the tension and let the muscles relax. Repeat 3 times.

EXERCISE – VI

Tighten the muscles of your feet and calves by stretching out legs and pointing toes away from you. Take a deep breath and hold tension for 5 seconds. Now breathe out and release the tension. Allow muscles of buttocks to relax. Repeat 3 times.

Make this physical relaxation a part of your daily routine.

All these exercises of relaxation are combined into a single relaxation posture known as Savasana

[b] SAVASANA (RELAXATION POSTURE)

Lie on your back, keep your hands by the side of thighs with palms facing upward. Keep legs apart and eyes closed. Concentrate on toes of both legs, slightly move them and relax. Now mentally disconnect yourself from this part of the body and feel that toes are completely relaxed. Now concentrate on the heels. Relax the heels and feel that they are relaxed. Concentrate on calf muscles, relax them. Feel that calf muscles of both legs are completely relaxed. Concentrate on knees. Concentrate on thighs and relax both thighs completely. Concentrate on hips, heavy bones and muscles.

Feel that hips and entire lower part of the body is completely relaxed. Once you relax a particular part you should not have any control over that part of body.

Concentrate on vertebral column. Relax the vertebral bones one by one. Slowly relax up to the neck. Then concentrate on stomach and relax the stomach muscles completely. Feel the movement of the abdomen due to slow breathing and relax it. Concentrate on chest and ribs. Relax chest and ribs. Breathe slowly and feel harmonious movement of lungs. Concentrate on shoulders. Relax shoulders, biceps, elbows, fore arms, wrist, palm and fingers. Concentrate on the neck, the entire weight of the head is over it. Relax it. Then concentrate on your head. Relax the head. Concentrate on face and relax face muscles. Concentrate on lips. Separate the lips slightly and relax. Separate two rows of teeth and relax them. Loosen your tongue and relax. Gently smile and relax your cheeks. Concentrate on nostrils, breathe slowly through nostrils and relax them. Concentrate on eyes, gently and slowly open the eyes partially. Look towards the roof of the sky and slowly close the eyes. The eyeball should be gently directed downwards. Relax eyeball and eyebrows. Feel that the entire region of the eye is completely relaxed. Concentrate on the forehead. Feel the entire forehead is relaxed. Concentrate on ears. Hear the sounds to come without resistance. Concentrate on the crown of the head. Relax the head fully. Relax your body fully. Feel that body is becoming lighter and it is floating in the space. Relax in this pose for a few minutes.

Inhale slowly and feel that all thes parts of the body are rejuvenating. Exhale and feel that all the impurities are going out.

With deep inhalation, raise both hands and place them above your head. Stretch your body from toes to the tip of the hand. Turn your entire body towards right. Stretch. Bring your body to the original position. Repeat the same process towards the left side. Slowly bring your hands by the side of the thighs. Slowly get up and sit for a few seconds and stand up.

[c] PRANAYAM

The next state in relaxation is the process of harmonizing the breath, the senses and the mind. It is called pranayam. By practicing pranayam, lungs get proper supply of oxygen and process of metabolism is carried out in an efficient manner. It steadies the mind in concentration.

Before practicing pranayam one should know correct method of breathing. Breathing through diaphragm has been discussed in para (a) of this section. Now we shall discuss breathing through chest.

- BREATHING THROUGH CHEST

This can be done in sitting position or lying down on the back. Breathe in deeply by expanding the chest. In this action the ribs will rise outwards. During breathing out exercise the ribs will contract inwards. Do not allow any movement of the stomach area.

Pranayam exercises should be preceded by savasana. So that body and mind are calm & undisturbed.

- DIRECTION FOR PRANAYAM
  - Pranayam should be done early in the morning after

Arthritis and Pain Management

intestine and urinary bladder is empty or it should be done after about four hours of taking food.
- Practice pranayam after yogic exercises and before meditation.
- The body should be in a relaxed state
- Pranayam should be done in airy and clean places.
- Sidhasana is the best posture for pranayam. However it can be done in Padmasana or Vajrasana poses also.

There are a number of types of pranayam but here we shall discuss only one type i.e. sukh purvaka pranayam (Easy comfortable breathing)

- ## SUKH PURVAKA PRANAYAM

Sit in comfortable position as per your convenience. Keep spine, neck and head erect. Keep middle and index fingers bent and other three stretched. Close right nostril with right thumb. Inhale slowly from the left nostril. Now close the left nostril with little and ring fingers of right hand, exhale slowly and harmoniously. Draw in air through the right nostril and exhale slowly through the left nostril. This completes one round. The ratio of inhalation and exhalation should be 1:2 i.e. inhale for 5 seconds and exhale for 10 seconds. During inhalation and exhalation expand and contract lungs as much as possible.

After three month of practice introduce retention of breath. The proper time of inhalation, retention and exhalation should be 1:2:2. In advance stage one may even practice the ratio 1:4:2. After inhalation slowly bend the neck and rest the chin on collarbone while retaining breath. Before exhalation slowly lift the head, keep it erect and then exhale.

The first symptom of correct practice of pranayam is that you should feel fresh. In case you feel the headache, heaviness and uneasiness, discontinue the retention of breath and consult an expert.

Last stage in relaxation is the meditation which is discussed below.

[d] MEDITATION

In these times the stress related illnesses are on the rise. We find conflict at the level of family, community, nation and the world. In order to escape stress and tension, people try a variety of methods i.e. some visit places of entertainment, some engage in sensual pleasure while the others turn to alcohol and drugs. However, these escape routes give only temporary happiness. However, if we read writings of saints through the ages, we find that true happiness and peace lies with in us.

During last few decades we find that more and more people are coming to the same conclusion that true happiness can be discovered within us and people are exploring meditation as a means of finding a way out of stress and tension. It has been demonstrated under scientific investigations that meditation improves hypertension, insomnia, chronic pain, asthma and anxiety. In meditation our body becomes totally relaxed. It is said that one hour of meditation is equal to four hours of sleep. We come out of meditation with renewed strength and vitality.

- **DIFFERENT STEPS IN MEDITATION**
  - **Time and place :** Meditation should be done at a time and place when, there is no disturbance. Slowly as we develop concentration, we can meditate even in noisy surroundings. The time between 3 to 6 o'clock in the morning is most appropriate for meditation when we are fully awake and relaxed.
  - **Selection of posture :** We should sit in posture, which is most convenient to us. Sukhasana, Padmasana and Vajrasana are some of the postures out of which the most convenient may be chosen. In case of orthopaedic problem one can practice meditation in sitting or even lying position with back straight.
  - **Concentration :** There are two stages of meditation. These are
    i. Constantly thinking on one object or thought to the exclusion of all others.
    ii. Keeping the mind free of all thoughts.

In the first stage, one should sit in a comfortable posture. Close the eyes and relax. One must concentrate on an object and engage in the repetition of mantra into which he has been initiated. When one starts repeating the mantra one comes to know the innumerable other thoughts which are submerged in one's subconscious mind and rise to conscious level and cause disturbance to the concentration on the mantra. When concentration to mantra along with the feeling of its meaning is increased through a long and continued practice, mind reaches a stage of meditation.

In the second stage, keep the ears open and let the external sounds impinge on them naturally. One should also witness the inner thoughts that arise one after another in an endless succession. One should not pay attention to either the external sounds or the inner thoughts. In the early stages care be taken not to go to sleep. By continuous practice for a long time the mind will become non-objectified.

Begin with 5 minutes and increase the time of meditation for thirty minutes and more.

❖ Step – 7

POSITIVE THINKING

The disease arthritis sets in the middle or later years of life. In this stage of life people consider themselves worn out, non-productive, unattractive and full of health problems. They feel sorry for themselves and expect others also to feel sorry for them. This self-pitying makes the situation worse. To change the circumstances, one should first start thinking differently.

When we reach up to the evening of life we become wise, experienced, emotionally matured and free from many responsibilities of upbringing children etc. These qualities and situations are enough to get real happiness. So, we should stop berating & depreciating ourselves. It is advisable not to look down on our problems, rather look up at them. Develop self-confidence and change the attitude towards life. We should divert our attention from feelings of pain and suffering and self-pitying thoughts by trying to keep busy in fruitful activities.

We often observe that pains, aches or any other disease aggravate at night. Why is it so? It is because at sleeping hours we have no other occupation except thinking or brooding about ourselves. I have myself noticed that when I go out or somebody drops in to chat, my sciatica pain evaporates, as if it was never there. So change the circumstances, go out and meet people, quit thinking constantly of yourself, think of others. Being self-centered aggravates the problem.

You can also take up a satisfying hobby to keep yourself busy. Get interested in something to forget the nagging pain. As you know that prolonged inactivity produces disability so fill your days with creative activity ad emphasize more on physical activity.

The level of mercury in our pain thermometer is directly proportional to our way of thinking. The negative thoughts like anger, hatred, jealousy, guilt, suspicion and anxiety impose negative influence on our body and actually upsets body rhythm with an increase in the feeling of pain.

The best fruitful way to keep yourself engaged is to go out and see how you can help people who are suffering more than you on account of poverty, disability or mental agony. You will find a great sense of achievement and lot of satisfaction in helping the needy. This positive approach will definitely ease your sufferings.

Whenever you are depressed, count the blessings God has bestowed on you. Try to find happiness in small things like blooming of a flower in the garden, smile of a child, freshness of breeze, chirping of birds etc. It is the best to try to look at the brighter side of the life and be optimistic.

❖ Step – 8

GETTING BACK TO NORMAL ACTIVITIES

The common characteristic of people with pain is that they restrict their physical as well as social activities. Some of them no longer go shopping, driving, playing, walking or playing with children or travelling in bus and train.

In order to get back to normal activities, the first step is to monitor yourself. Record information about the time spent by you on lying down, reclining, sitting, walking, eating, cooking, taking bath, reading, watching T.V., meeting friends, playing with children and other activities. Recording this information for two to three days will give you an idea about how you spend your time. If you are locked in chronic pain, you will see that you are spending more time on reclining and lying down. In such a condition, the muscles will lose tone and become weak. The pain, which originated in one part of body will become generalized giving feeling of bruising, stiffness and discomfort throughout the day. Therefore while returning to any activity after a long time, there is a need to progressively prepare the muscles. A person in pain needs to be helped to cope with fear and anxiety arising out of increasing mobility.

The strategies outlined here assume that you are not very active. To start with, select an activity you have neglected for long. Set yourself a target, which you think is comfortable for you. Progressively increase the target. Sitting and walking are basic to most of the activities hence we shall discuss them in detail.

- *SITTING*

In case you are accustomed to reclining and lying, your muscles would have been weakened. You have to start with sitting position and learn to sit still.

Find a chair, which should support you completely from head through back, your buttocks and thighs. Sit with your bottom well back and spine straight, feet firmly on floor and hands resting on your thighs or on arms of the chair. This is a comfortable sitting position.

Start breathing slowly through diaphragm. Set a target for yourself. In case you are accustomed to reclining and lying, you may start with a target of 5 minutes. Aim to sit for 5 minutes irrespective of comfort or discomfort. Progressively, increase your time of sitting each day. You can have more than one session of sitting each day. As you increase the time of sitting in one session, you can add some pleasurable activity. Use relaxation tape to extend your sitting time.

Remember, relaxation and diaphragmatic breathing is key to sitting comfortably. Within a week or two, you would be in a position to sit with break for exercise, meals etc from 9 a.m. to 5 p.m. You may now decide to visit a neighbour for a cup of tea. However, decide in advance as to how long you will stay. Tell your friend and leave at a pre-arranged time. Do not make a mistake to sit longer as you are feeling comfortable. In such a case you may be overwhelmed by pain and discomfort later.

After one adventure, plan the next and you may now go to a restaurant for lunch/dinner. It usually takes about an hour and a half, so make it a target. You may feel pain when you get back home but do not make it an excuse not to do it again. Plan your social life and plan for success. Do not be discouraged by set backs but start all over again.

- **WALKING**

    Walking is central to most of the activities. Walking strengthens leg muscles, back muscles and helps in circulation. Confidence in walking is important to social and other essential tasks. If a person spends lot of time reclining or lying down, his muscles will not be strong enough for long distance walking. Progressive exercises are essential for getting fit for walking. It is possible that a person in this condition will experience pain after walking a short distance initially.

    Initially choose a flat and even terrain for walking. Wear shoes, which have thick cushion in the soles. And wear a good pair of cotton socks. Wear light clothing.

    On the first occasion plan to walk not more than 5 minutes or say 40-50 m. Aim to succeed on this first occasion by setting a time limit or distance limit. Repeat it on three occasions.

    Now set progressively higher target say 8 minutes and increase it to 10 minutes next time. Repeat each target on three occasions. While walking enjoy the scenery, enjoy the fresh air and enjoy the surroundings. In case you feel pain do relaxation and breathing through diaphragm. Relaxation should be done before and after the walk.

    Progressively increase your time of walking. Be adventurous in terms of walking even though you may feel some

Arthritis and Pain Management

discomfort. When you start walking 30 minutes, you would be walking even farther than an average pain free individual. Be proud of yourself. A brisk walking of half an hour a day will do a lot of good to you as walking increases general fitness, stimulates the release of endorphins and hence reduces pain.

After sitting and walking exercises, one can start the right type of yogic exercises as given in chapter 2.6.

❖ **Step – 9**

GETTING BACK TO WORK

Untreated or badly treated chronic pain reduces one's capacity to work. However, by proper treatment people can be helped back to some kind of successful working life. The different steps involved are: -

- Reducing pain
- Increasing mobility
- Sustaining effort for longer time
- Achieving better quality of life.
- Changing attitude towards employment
- Need for training/retraining.

There is a sense of panic about losing a job and your sole purpose of getting better becomes to get back to your work as quickly as possible. However, it is not always possible to resume your normal employment due to physical as well as legal reasons. When planning to get back to work increase your mobility and stamina to the level that you can spend at least 2-3 hours on any job continuously i.e. build yourself physically to cope with the work you are planning to do. Accept your limitations and avoid competition with physically Stronger people.

Take pride in stepping away from the disabled status. Progressive training with small increase in activity is very important. Build up slowly but surely. In case you are not able to get back to your previous work, think about re-training in something less exciting. In order to get distraction from pain, find a way of becoming occupied in an absorbing task as it will give you a purpose of life.

❖ Step – 10

COPING WITH A SET BACK

Setbacks, relapses and pain flare-ups are inevitable in arthritis. These set backs sometimes threaten the rehabilitation for some people. It is important to anticipate how these setbacks occur and device ways to cope with them. The setbacks usually occur due to overstrain i.e. trying to compete with normal people, trying to accomplish too large a task or setting goal which is much higher than the stage of rehabilitation.

Setbacks are common and usually people indulge in negative thoughts after setbacks. They start saying to themselves 'I will never get better'. It is going to be worse in future. What is wrong with me? What have I done to deserve this? Etc. It is important to recognize that if you have chronic pain, you are likely to get setbacks in the beginning of the treatment and it is likely that you will be discouraged and even be depressed. Begin to monitor your progress i.e. identify progress and measure the setbacks against the progress made. Make a diary and note down information regarding frequency and intensity of pain, the factors, which increase the pain such as anxiety, tension etc., the factors that reduce pain such as relaxation, listening to music, holidays, meeting friends etc. Also note down specific situations in which pain is experienced or aggravated.

If you have data as a result of on going monitoring you will see for yourself that progress is in fact being made. You may even ask a friend or family member to remind you as to what your condition was before you started your recovery. You will find that change may be appreciable at a time in at least one or more areas of observation such as reduction of frequency of pain, reduction in intensity or duration of pain or it may result in reduction in the amount of medication required to control pain.

You have to accept that setbacks are a part of normal experience and they should not be treated as a catastrophe. Accept that setback is a price you have to pay for doing something enjoyable and exciting. Take corrective measures and develop a routine of thinking and behavior which will quickly bring you back to normal state. After a series of tests and exercises one can reduce the physical exercises till one gets back to normal. Learn from experience and device new and better ways of coping with these setbacks.

❖ **Step – 11**

DOCTOR AS A FRIEND

A person with chronic pain is not generally in such an emotional state that he can choose between different options. He tends to rely on the doctor for diagnosis of disease and the treatment and becomes a passive recipient of medical care. Regarding medical consultations, the doctor prescribes medicines and gives an assurance that there is no life threatening illness or disorder. This message may be interpreted differently and he may infer that either the doctor is withholding some bad news or implies that there is nothing wrong physically and therefore the pain is imaginary. This type of misunderstanding may result in breakdown of faith in the doctor and communication with him.

In case one is having a chronic pain, he has to change his approach to medical consultations. Seek doctor's advice about increasing mobility and strength, and involve him in planning for your future well being.

In case your doctor is proposing investigations and treatment with drugs without discussion, ask questions on the following points.

- Reasons for investigation
- Name of the drug
- What is it for? whether it is a painkiller, tranquilizer, muscle relaxant or anti depressant.
- How much and how often should it be taken?
- How long is it required?
- What are its short term and long term side effects?
- Inform him about other medicines being taken by you. How will this medicine react to them?
- If medicine is withdrawn what will be the effect?

After taking medication for few days, find out the effect of medicine and in case you are not happy about the effect of medicines, discuss with him about changing the same.

Do not suddenly stop taking medicine without consulting the doctor. Doctor will know how to reduce the dosage safely & systematically.

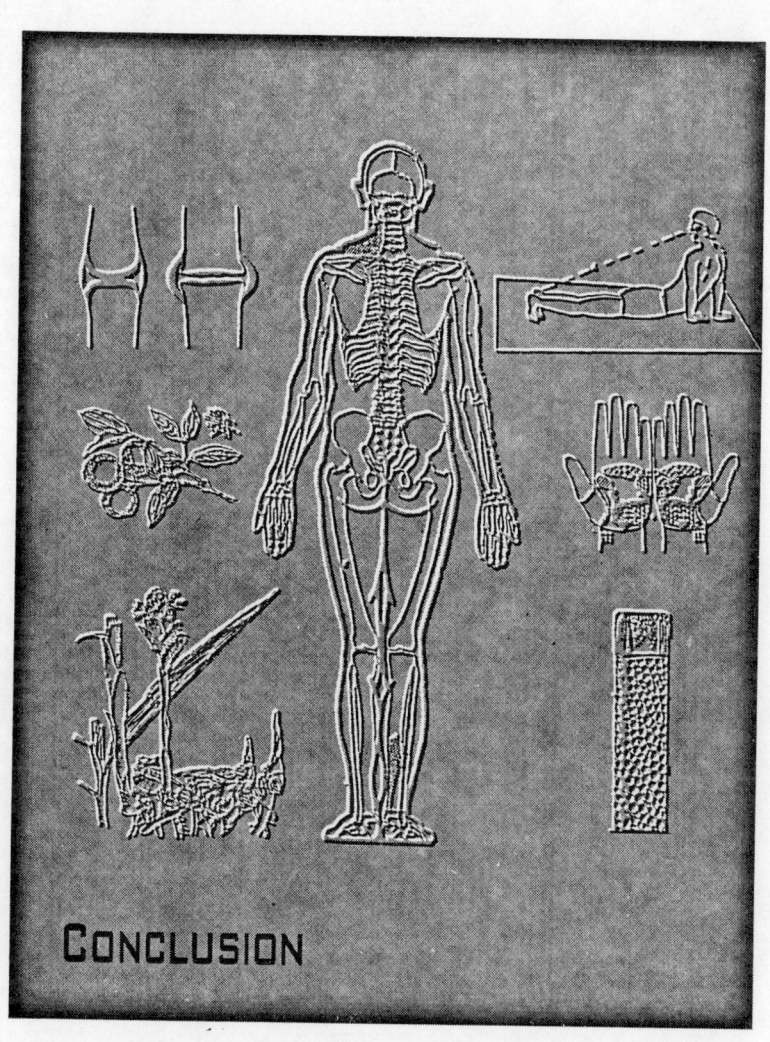

CONCLUSION

Chapter

4

CONCLUSION

Healing does not mean that since the body has malfunctioned there should be some underlying physical cause that must be found out and corrected. When the body malfunctions, it has an effect on us at various levels. In a holistic approach the treatment should not be confined to the physical cause alone but to the person as a whole. In order to achieve true healing the body and mind should work together. Whatever therapy we may choose, it can only be effective if we have faith in the healing system and the person who helps us heal ourselves.

Descartes said " I consider human body as a machine. My thought compares the sick man and an ill made clock with my idea of a healthy man and a well made clock." This dualism is the basis of modern medicine that fails to take into account mind body relationship in the healing process.

It should be mentioned here that we cannot ignore the technological advances made in allopathy. Further, without complementary support from allopathic system for diagnostics and follow up tests, there is little that an alternative system of medicine can achieve. There is therefore a need that research in alternative systems of medicine be encouraged and medical students in allopathy are exposed to these systems of medicine also.

As we have already discussed, there is chronic pain in joints in case of arthritis. Besides, there is inflammation and stiffness. The pain is severe at times while it is dull at other times but it reminds its presence all the time. There is no magic cure of the disease as yet. However, there are enormous commercial interests supplying services and products to cure the pain. This raises hopes and as a result you could spend a fortune trying to find a cure, which might not be there. Taking advantage of your helplessness even some doctors may start prescribing steroids indiscriminately which in short run reduces pain dramatically but have dangerous side effects. It is therefore necessary to warn you about all this. You may not be able to spend money on a large scale for life so think of some simple remedies to ease your discomfort.

Heat is a source of comfort in pain as it promotes circulation. In order to provide localized warmth one can use infrared lamp or even warm water bottle. In some cases ice pack wrapped in a cloth will be very relaxing. One may experiment with warm as well as cold packs and find out what is most suitable for him.

Take action at the first sign of the onset of pain instead of increasing your tension and subsequently pain. Take a mild painkiller and relax. Depending on the type of pain and how it is ameliorated or aggravated one can also take an appropriate homeopathic medicine. Acupressure is also a very effective tool in controlling and managing pain.

Conclusion

There are a number of similarities between various healing systems discussed in this book. It is up to the doctor within us to harness the healing force in order to achieve a balance between body and mind.

The holistic approach to healthcare is the new mantra of this millennium. This approach is based on the principal that human organism is multidimensional, consisting of body and mind. The disease results from an imbalance from within or from an external source. The human body possesses a powerful capacity to heal itself by bringing different forces in a state of equilibrium. The primary task of a medical practitioner is to encourage and assist the patient in his attempt to heal himself.

In order to begin the process of healing, first and the foremost thing is that you should have the willpower to get well. Hence, do not allow your doctor or anybody else to take full responsibility of your health and well being as they can only offer specific treatments for specific problems but cannot cause miracles. Take steps to work on the management of your own pain and your ultimate rehabilitation.